About the NCCN Guidelines for Patients®

National Comprehensive Cancer Network®

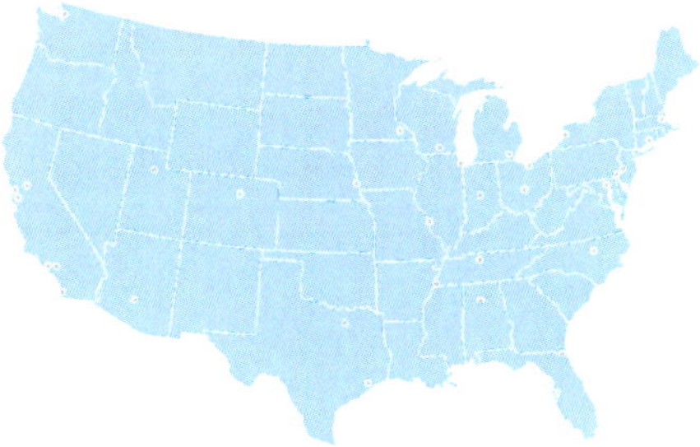

Did you know that top cancer centers across the United States work together to improve cancer care? This alliance of leading cancer centers is called the National Comprehensive Cancer Network® (NCCN®).

Cancer care is always changing. NCCN develops evidence-based cancer care recommendations used by health care providers worldwide. These frequently updated recommendations are the NCCN Clinical Practice Guidelines in Oncology (NCCN Guidelines®). The NCCN Guidelines for Patients plainly explain these expert recommendations for people with cancer and caregivers.

These NCCN Guidelines for Patients are based on the NCCN Clinical Practice Guidelines in Oncology (NCCN Guidelines®) for Non-Small Cell Lung Cancer, Version 3.2025 – January 14, 2025.

Learn how the NCCN Guidelines for Patients are developed
NCCN.org/patient-guidelines-process

View the NCCN Guidelines for Patients free online
NCCN.org/patientguidelines

Find an NCCN Cancer Center near you
NCCN.org/cancercenters

Connect with us

Supporters

NATIONAL COMPREHENSIVE CANCER NETWORK®
NCCN FOUNDATION
Guiding Treatment. Changing Lives.

NCCN Guidelines for Patients are supported by funding from the NCCN Foundation®

NCCN Foundation gratefully acknowledges the following corporate supporters for helping to make available these NCCN Guidelines for Patients: AbbVie; Boehringer Ingelheim Pharmaceuticals, Inc.; Daiichi Sankyo; Janssen Biotech, Inc.; Novocure; and Regeneron Pharmaceuticals, Inc.

NCCN independently adapts, updates, and hosts the NCCN Guidelines for Patients. Our corporate supporters do not participate in the development of the NCCN Guidelines for Patients and are not responsible for the content and recommendations contained therein.

To make a gift or learn more, visit online or email

NCCNFoundation.org/Donate

PatientGuidelines@NCCN.org

Contents

4 About early and locally advanced NSCLC

8 Lung nodules and cancer

19 Testing for early and locally advanced NSCLC

27 Improving life with supportive care

32 Planning primary treatment

41 Lung cancer surgery

53 Radiation therapy

58 Chemoradiation

63 Survivorship care

69 Other resources

73 Words to know

77 NCCN Contributors

78 NCCN Cancer Centers

80 Index

NCCN Foundation seeks to support the millions of patients and their families affected by a cancer diagnosis by funding and distributing NCCN Guidelines for Patients. NCCN Foundation is also committed to advancing cancer treatment by funding the nation's promising doctors at the center of innovation in cancer research. For more details and the full library of patient and caregiver resources, visit NCCN.org/patients.

National Comprehensive Cancer Network (NCCN) and NCCN Foundation
3025 Chemical Road, Suite 100, Plymouth Meeting, PA 19462 USA

1

About early and locally advanced NSCLC

5 What are early and locally advanced NSCLCs?

6 How are these lung cancers found?

6 How are these lung cancers treated?

7 What can you do to get the best care?

Non-small cell lung cancer (NSCLC) is the most common type of lung cancer. Early and locally advanced cancers haven't spread far from the lung. There are several treatments that may cure or control the growth of these cancers.

What are early and locally advanced NSCLCs?

Early and locally advanced non-small cell lung cancers (NSCLCs) affect certain types of lung cells that have grown from the airways into other lung tissue but haven't spread to other organs.

This description is important because treatment differs between lung cancer types and where lung cancer is in the body.

Types of NSCLC

NSCLC is a group of cancers. Each cancer in this group affects a different type of lung cell.

You have NSCLC if you have one of these cancers:

- Lung adenocarcinoma (A-deh-noh-KAR-sih-NOH-muh) affects lung cells that make mucus.
- Large cell carcinoma (kar-sin-OH-ma) of the lung forms from large cells in the airways.
- Squamous (squay-mous) cell carcinoma of the lung affects protective cells that line the airways.

There are more types of NSCLC, but they are much less common. And some lung cancers are a mix of cell types.

Early and locally advanced sites

NSCLC affects the cells that line the airways of the lung. Cancer causes these cells to grow out of control and form a tumor on the wall of the airway.

Tumor growth into other tissue

Early and locally advanced NSCLCs have grown through the wall of the airway and into other lung tissue.

Some of these cancers have also grown into the wall of the lung or through the lung wall into other tissue.

Possible spread to nearby lymph nodes

Locally advanced NSCLC sometimes has spread to lymph nodes inside the lung or within the chest. Lymph nodes are small bean-shaped structures that fight disease.

No spread to other organs

Early and locally advanced NSCLCs have not spread to the fluid within the lining around the lung or formed tumors inside the lining. They also have not spread to the other lung or to another organ.

How are these lung cancers found?

Many times, early and locally advanced NSCLC is found by accident. A scan for another health issue may reveal a spot that could be cancer. Learn how a team of experts discovers if a spot is cancer in *Chapter 2: Lung nodules and cancer.*

How are these lung cancers treated?

Surgery is often used to remove early and locally advanced NSCLC but is not the only option. There's no single treatment plan that's best for everyone.

Testing is needed to plan treatment

Your care team will give tests to learn the type of lung cancer you have and where the cancer is in your body. They will also test for important cancer features called biomarkers. Tests needed to plan treatment are described in *Chapter 3: Testing for early and locally advanced NSCLC.*

Supportive care addresses the challenges of cancer

Supportive care involves multiple types of aid that improve quality of life. It includes care to prevent and relieve symptoms. More information is in *Chapter 4: Improving life with supportive care.*

Confused about lung cancer?

People use the term lung cancer to describe many cancers. Sometimes, they misuse the term, so here's an explanation of what lung cancer is and what it isn't.

What lung cancer is

Simply, lung cancer causes uncontrolled growth of lung cells. There are many types of cells in the lungs, so there are many types of lung cancer.

Non-small cell lung cancer (NSCLC) is the most common type of lung cancer. So when people talk about lung cancer, they're likely talking about NSCLC.

This book is part of a 2-book series on NSCLC. There are NCCN Guidelines for Patients on other types of lung cancers.

What is not lung cancer

Cancers that have spread to the lungs are not lung cancers. For example, stomach cancer that has spread to the lungs is still stomach cancer. Treatment for cancers that have spread to the lungs is discussed in the guidelines for that cancer type.

The library of NCCN Guidelines for Patients can be found at NCCN.org/patientguidelines and on the NCCN Patient Guides for Cancer app.

Cancer staging is essential for planning treatment

A cancer stage is a rating of the growth and spread of lung cancer. Learn about treatment options based on cancer staging in *Chapter 5: Planning primary treatment.*

Multiple treatments often are used to get the best results

Treatment results can be improved when other types of treatment are used with surgery. The types and order of treatments are explained in *Chapter 6: Lung cancer surgery.*

If you can't have surgery, there are other good options. Some early cancers are cured with radiation therapy as discussed in *Chapter 7: Radiation therapy.* Other cancers are treated with 2 different types of therapies, which are described in *Chapter 8: Chemoradiation.*

What can you do to get the best care?

Advocate for yourself. You have an important role to play in your care. In fact, you're more likely to get the care you want by asking questions and making shared decisions with your care team.

The NCCN Guidelines for Patients will help you understand cancer care. With better understanding, you'll be more prepared to discuss your care with your team and share your concerns. Many people feel more satisfied when they play an active role in their care.

Why you should read this book

Making decisions about cancer care can be stressful. You may need to make tough decisions under pressure about complex choices.

The NCCN Guidelines for Patients are trusted by patients and providers. They clearly explain current care recommendations made by respected experts in the field. Recommendations are based on the latest research and practices at leading cancer centers.

Cancer care is not the same for everyone. By following expert recommendations for your situation, you are more likely to improve your care and have better outcomes as a result. Use this book as your guide to find the information you need to make important decisions.

You may not know what to ask your care team. That's common. Each chapter in this book ends with an important section called *Questions to ask.* These suggested questions will help you get more information on all aspects of your care.

Take the next step and keep reading to learn what is the best care for you!

2
Lung nodules and cancer

9 Lung nodule experts

10 Risk factors for lung cancer

11 Signs of lung cancer on imaging

12 Planning follow-up testing

12 Types of follow-up testing

13 Follow-up testing for solid nodules

14 Follow-up testing for subsolid nodules

15 Making a plan to remove tissue

16 Removing samples to test for cancer

16 Confirming lung cancer

17 What's next?

18 Key points

18 Questions to ask

Many people have small masses of tissue in their lungs, called nodules. Lung nodules are sometimes found by chance. This chapter explains the next steps of care when these nodules could be cancer.

Lung nodule experts

A nodule is a small mass of tissue that can grow inside your lung. Most lung nodules are not cancer and are harmless. These nodules may be caused by infections, scar tissue, or other health conditions.

When a nodule found by chance seems to be cancer, it takes a team of experts to decide the best course of care.

Your care team should consist of members from different fields of medicine, including the following board-certified specialists:

- A **pulmonologist** is an expert in lung diseases.
- A **thoracic radiologist** is an expert in imaging of the chest. Imaging takes pictures of the inside of the body.
- A **thoracic surgeon** is an expert in operations within the chest.

To decide if a nodule is cancer, your team will:

- Assess how likely the nodule is cancer by reviewing your risk factors for lung cancer and the results of your imaging
- Request more imaging if there may be cancer
- If needed, perform a procedure, called a biopsy, to test the nodule for cancer

Lung nodule

A lung nodule is a small mass of tissue in the lung. Many people have lung nodules. Most are not cancer. When nodules are found by imaging, you may receive more scans to assess if the nodule is cancer.

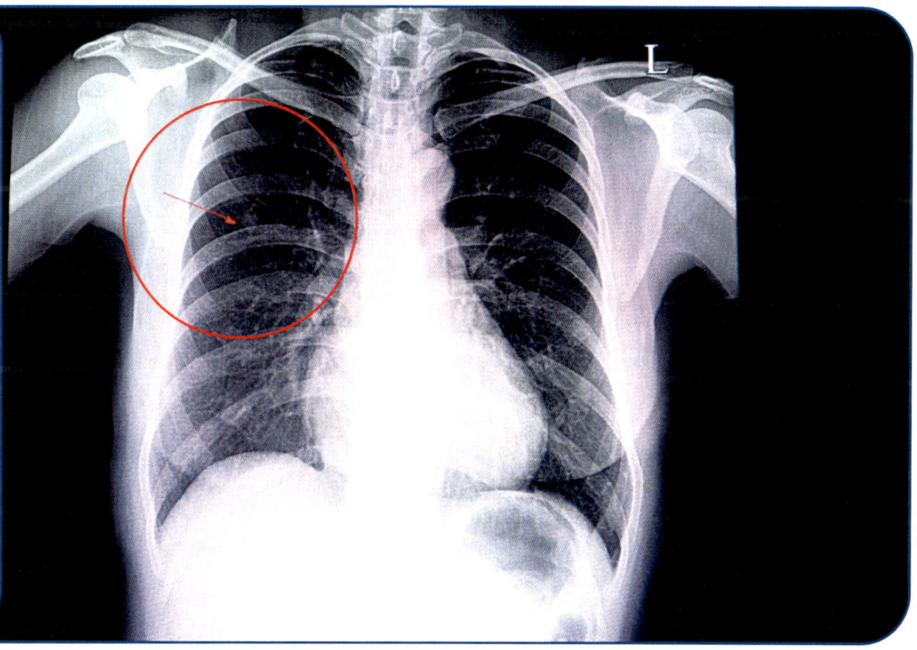

Risk factors for lung cancer

To help decide if more testing of the nodule is needed, your care team will assess your risk for lung cancer by asking you about known risk factors.

Tobacco smoke

The biggest risk factor for lung cancer is smoking tobacco. Tobacco smoke contains more than 50 compounds known to cause cancer. The risk grows the more times a person smokes and the longer they smoke.

Even if you don't smoke, exposure to second-hand smoke increases the risk of lung cancer. Secondhand smoke is the smoke exhaled by another person and the smoke from the burning end of tobacco products.

Cancer-causing agents

You're more likely to get lung cancer, especially if you smoke, after exposure to:

- Radon
- Asbestos
- Arsenic, beryllium, cadmium, chromium, and nickel
- Coal smoke, soot, silica, and diesel fumes
- Air pollution by fine particulates, ozone, nitrogen oxides, and sulfur dioxide

Age

As you age, you are more likely to get lung cancer. In recent years, half of the people diagnosed with lung cancer were over 71 years of age. Only 6 out of 100 people with lung cancer were under the age of 55 years at the time of diagnosis.

Previous cancers and cancer treatment

The risk for lung cancer increases after having some types of cancer:

- Having one type of lung cancer increases your risk for other types of lung cancers.
- If you had lymphoma, you are more likely to get lung cancer.

Who gets lung cancer?

Experts are still learning why one person gets lung cancer and another does not.

We know some of the risk factors that increase a person's chance for getting lung cancer.

Yet people with many risk factors may never get lung cancer, and people with no risk factors sometimes get lung cancer.

Despite smoking being the biggest risk factor, the number of people who do not smoke but are getting lung cancer is rising worldwide. More research is needed to learn what are the risk factors of lung cancer in this group.

- If you've had another smoking-related cancer, such as head and neck cancer, your risk for lung cancer is increased.

Some cancer treatments also increase the risk of getting lung cancer years after treatment, including:

- Radiation therapy to the chest, especially if you smoke
- Treatment of Hodgkin lymphoma with an alkylating cancer drug

Family history of lung cancer

Your risk for lung cancer is increased if your birth parent, sibling, or child has had lung cancer. Your risk is even higher if lung cancer occurred at a young age or among multiple relatives.

Other lung diseases

Some lung diseases can increase the risk of lung cancer. There's a strong link between lung cancer and these diseases:

- Chronic obstructive pulmonary disease (COPD), which causes lung damage or too much mucus
- Pulmonary fibrosis, which is major scarring of lung tissue

Signs of lung cancer on imaging

Your radiologist will assess if the nodule may be cancer by reviewing your imaging. Important results are the features of the nodule, abnormal lung tissue, and hot spots.

Features of the nodule

Nodules caused by cancer have specific features. They aren't likely to have calcium and compared to nodules without cancer, often have these features:

- Rough edges and odd shapes
- Fast growth and large size
- High density

Abnormal lung tissue

Besides nodules, imaging may show other abnormal findings in the lungs. It may show tissue inflammation and tissue scarring.

Hot spots

If you had a positron emission tomography (PET) scan, your radiologist will look for hot (or bright) spots.

Before the scan, a tracer was injected into one of your veins. Cancer cells take in more of injected tracer than normal cells and appear as hot spots on the images.

Cancer is not the only health condition to produce hots spots, so the cause often needs to be confirmed by other testing.

Planning follow-up testing

Based on your risk factors and the imaging results, your care team will make a follow-up plan specific to you.

NCCN recommendations for follow-up testing are explained on the next pages. They are grouped by nodule density:

- **Solid nodules** are dense.
- **Subsolid nodules** may have a mix of high and low density or have only low density.

The nodule size is also very important for planning, which is measured in millimeters (mm). To picture the size of your nodule, compare its size to the tip of a new crayon. The tip of a crayon is about 2 mm.

To understand NCCN recommendations, the types of follow-up tests are explained next as well as the reasoning for the tests.

Types of follow-up testing

There are 3 types of follow-up tests for lung nodules:

- A computed tomography (CT) scan is a more detailed kind of x-ray that shows the density and size of nodules.
- A PET/CT scan can detect small amounts of cancer that CT missed.
- A biopsy is a procedure that removes a small amount of tissue or fluid for cancer testing. It's the only way to confirm, or diagnose, cancer.

Why get scans instead of a biopsy?

Scans are less invasive than a biopsy. Your team wants to see clear signs of cancer on imaging scans before doing a biopsy.

CT scans

You may get low-dose CT or a diagnostic CT of the chest. NCCN experts prefer low-dose CT for cancer screening unless a clearer image is needed.

Low-dose CT uses much less radiation than a diagnostic scan. It also does not require contrast, which is a substance that makes clearer images.

Often, one CT scan doesn't clearly show whether a nodule is cancer. Instead, CT needs to be repeated over time to find signs of cancer.

PET/CT scan

A PET/CT scan after a chest CT scan may find cancer quicker than repeated CT scans. It is also useful for showing signs of cancer spreading in the body.

Your whole body will be scanned, or the scan will extend from above your neck down to the middle of your thighs.

Why get a biopsy instead of scans?

If your team strongly suspects cancer, a biopsy may save time by allowing you to start cancer treatment earlier than if you had a series of scans.

Follow-up testing for solid nodules

NCCN recommendations for follow-up testing of solid nodules are listed in **Guide 1**.

Follow-up testing is partly based on your risk for lung cancer. Your risk is low if you have minor or no risk factors. You must not have smoked or smoked very little.

Solid nodules smaller than 6 mm in size don't need immediate follow-up testing. Your team will decide what care is needed.

Nodules between 6 mm and 8 mm in size will be checked between 6 to 12 months, and if you have a high risk for lung cancer, checked a second time between 18 to 24 months after the first scan.

Nodules that are bigger than 8 mm may be checked with CT in 3 months or with PET/CT now, or they may be biopsied.

Guide 1
Follow-up testing for solid lung nodules

Low risk for lung cancer	**Nodule is smaller than 6 mm**	No routine follow-up testing is needed. Your team will decide the next steps of care.
	Nodule is between 6 and 8 mm	A CT scan is recommended at 6 to 12 months after the first scan. If there is no increase in nodule size or density, you may get another CT scan at 18 to 24 months after the first scan.
	Nodule is larger than 8 mm	There are 3 options: • CT scan in 3 months • PET/CT scan now • Biopsy now
High risk for lung cancer	**Nodule is smaller than 6 mm**	It is an option to get a CT scan at 12 months after the first scan. If there is no increase in nodule size or density, your team will decide the next steps of care.
	Nodule is between 6 and 8 mm	A CT scan is recommended at 6 to 12 months and again at 18 to 24 months after the first scan.
	Nodule is larger than 8 mm	There are 3 options: • CT scan in 3 months • PET/CT scan now • Biopsy now

Follow-up testing for subsolid nodules

Subsolid nodules include non-solid nodules and part-solid nodules.

- Non-solid nodules have low density and are also called ground-glass opacities or ground-glass nodules.
- Part-solid nodules have both high and low areas of density.

Many subsolid nodules go away in time without treatment. Those that remain are not likely to become a problem.

Follow-up testing for subsolid nodules is listed in **Guide 2**.

One subsolid nodule smaller than 6 mm does not need routine follow-up testing. Larger or multiple nodules will be checked again.

Guide2
Follow-up testing for subsolid lung nodules

1 non-solid nodule	**Nodule is smaller than 6 mm**	No routine follow-up testing is needed. Your team will decide the next steps of care.
	Nodule is 6 mm or larger	A CT scan is recommended at 6 to 12 months after the first scan. If there is no increase in nodule size or density, repeat CT every 2 years until 5 years after the first scan.
1 part-solid nodule	**Nodule is smaller than 6 mm**	No routine follow-up testing is needed. Your team will decide the next steps of care.
	Nodule is 6 mm or larger	A CT scan is recommended at 3 to 6 months after the first scan. If there's no nodule growth and the solid part remains smaller than 6 mm, repeat CT every year for 5 years. If the solid part is 6 mm or larger, you may get a PET/CT scan or a biopsy.
2 or more non-solid or part-solid nodules	**Nodules are smaller than 6 mm**	A CT scan is recommended at 3 to 6 months after the first scan of the nodule. If there is no increase in nodule size or density, your team may want another CT at 2 and 4 years after the first scan.
	Nodules are 6 mm or larger	A CT scan is recommended at 3 to 6 months after the first scan. The next steps depend on the nodule that is the most likely to be cancer.

A single non-solid nodule larger than 6 mm will be checked at 6 to 12 months after the first scan. Nodules that are more likely to be cancer will be checked at 3 to 6 months. If a follow-up CT scan shows signs of cancer, you may get a PET/CT scan or biopsy.

Making a plan to remove tissue

If cancer is likely, tissue needs to be removed and tested. The plan to remove tissue differs among people. A plan that is best for you may not be the best plan for someone else.

When planning, your team will think about the size and location of tumors, your health history, and their experience. They rely on the results of a physical exam and imaging.

Your team will decide the best method

Removing tissue for cancer testing is not always easy. Your team will decide the best method to remove tissue. Ways to remove samples are described in the next section.

Your team may diagnose and stage the cancer at the same time

Cancer staging is a rating of the extent of cancer in the body. If scans showed multiple areas of cancer, the body part farthest from the lung nodule will be sampled and tested.

Your team will decide the best time for cancer testing

The decision of when to test for cancer is partly based on whether you will have surgical treatment or not.

Testing when surgery is not planned

Lung nodules that can't be fully removed by surgery are tested before cancer treatment starts. Surgery may not be a treatment option because of your overall health, location of a lung nodule, or advanced cancer.

Testing when surgery is planned

When nodules will be surgically treated, cancer testing may be done before or on the day of surgical treatment.

Cancer testing can be delayed for tiny nodules that are very likely to be early-stage lung cancer. Cancer testing done in advance of surgery would increase health risks, time spent, and costs. More lung tissue may be removed if the nodule is cancer.

There are times when it is better to diagnose before surgical treatment:

- You shouldn't wait until surgery if your care team strongly suspects a disease other than lung cancer.
- Early testing is also needed if whole-body drug treatment, called systemic therapy, will be received before surgery or if you will have a type of radiation therapy called stereotactic ablative radiotherapy.

Removing samples to test for cancer

Your team will choose a method that removes tissue that likely has cancer. They will consider the risk and ease of methods and what method you prefer.

- **External needle biopsies** involve guiding a thin needle through your skin and into the tumor. These procedures include transthoracic needle aspiration, core needle biopsies, pericardiocentesis, and thoracentesis.
- **Down-the-throat biopsies** involve guiding thin tools down your throat into your airways (bronchus) or food pipe (esophagus). These procedures include many types of bronchoscopy.
- **Keyhole surgeries** involve making small openings into your chest. Small tools are inserted through the holes to remove tissue. Compared to open surgery, this method is less invasive, which means healing is easier. These surgeries include mediastinoscopy and thoracoscopy. Thoracoscopy can be performed by video-assisted thoracoscopic surgery or robot-assisted thoracoscopic surgery.
- **Open surgery** involves making a large cut through your chest wall to remove tissue. Open surgery is seldom needed for diagnosis. You may have open surgery when other methods won't work or a larger piece of tissue is needed.

A pathologist is an expert in tissue and cells and confirming cancer. At some cancer centers, the pathologist checks the tissue size right away because it must be large enough to run several tests. This in-person method is called rapid on-site evaluation. It helps to prevent having the same procedure a second time.

Confirming lung cancer

A pathologist will prepare and then look at the tissue with a microscope. This takes a few days. The remaining tissue will be saved for possible future testing.

If non-small cell lung cancer (NSCLC) is found, the pathologist will identify the type:

- Adenocarcinoma is a cancer of cells that often line the air sacs in the lungs and make mucus. This is the most common type of NSCLC.
- Large cell carcinoma is a cancer of cells that are large in size compared to other cells in the airways.
- Squamous cell carcinoma is a cancer of thin, flat cells that protect the airways.
- There are also rare and mixed types of NSCLC.

The results of lab tests used for diagnosis are recorded in a pathology report.

What's next?

The next steps of care are based on whether cancer was found in the biopsy samples. Read the section that matches your test results.

The nodule was not cancer

Even if no cancer was found, your team may refer you for lung cancer screening. Lung cancer screening is for people at high risk for lung cancer. For more information, read the *NCCN Guidelines for Patients: Lung Cancer Screening.*

Researchers are studying ways to prevent lung cancer caused by smoking. Treatments to prevent cancer are called chemopreventive agents. There may be a clinical trial on preventing lung cancer that you could join.

The nodule is cancer

Your team will need to learn more about you and the cancer.

This book focuses on early and locally advanced NSCLC. We discuss what tests your team needs to plan treatment in Chapter *3: Testing for early and locally NSCLC*.

If you were diagnosed with a cancer other than NSCLC, search the library of NCCN of Guidelines for Patients for treatment information.

The library of NCCN Guidelines for Patients can be found at NCCN.org/patientguidelines and on the NCCN Patient Guides for Cancer app.

"Don't Google your diagnosis and assume that statistics define your life! Every person's cancer and situation is different."

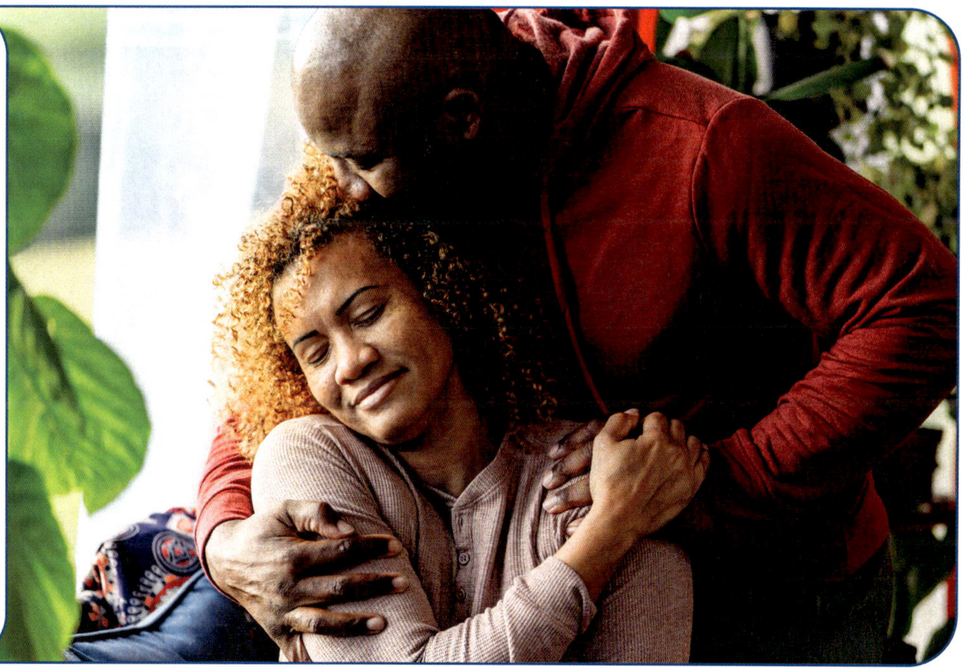

Key points

- It takes a team of experts to assess lung nodules for cancer.
- Tobacco smoking is the biggest but not the only risk factor for lung cancer.
- Signs of lung cancer can be found with imaging of the chest.
- Lung nodule experts assess changes in a nodule with a series of CT scans over time. Nodules that quickly increase in size or density are more likely to be cancer.
- If the nodule is likely cancer, you may have a PET/CT scan, or nodule samples may be removed and tested for cancer.

Questions to ask

- How did you decide what type of follow-up testing is needed for the lung nodule?
- What type of procedures will be done to remove and store tissue samples for future testing?
- Do I need to start lung cancer screening? Is there a clinical trial on preventing lung cancer that I can join?
- What type of cancer do I have?

3

Testing for early and locally advanced NSCLC

20 Team evaluation

20 First set of tests

22 Tests before treatment

25 What's next?

26 Key points

26 Questions to ask

Your care team will make a treatment plan just for you. To make the plan, they'll need to learn about the lung cancer and your general health. This chapter describes the tests needed for treatment planning.

Team evaluation

It takes a team to plan treatment of non-small cell lung cancer (NSCLC). If more than one type of treatment is an option, your team will consist of members from different fields of medicine, such as:

- A **thoracic surgical oncologist** is an expert in removing cancer from the chest.
- A **radiation oncologist** is an expert in treating cancer with radiation.
- A **medical oncologist** is an expert in treating cancer with drugs.

Many people also have team members that provide supportive care, which is discussed in *Chapter 4: Improving life with supportive care.*

You are also an important part of the team. Your participation is as important as that of any specialist on your team.

First set of tests

After confirming lung cancer, your team will want to learn more about the cancer and you.

They need to know about your general health and well-being. They also need to find out the extent of the lung cancer in your body. This is called staging the cancer.

The first set of tests needed to learn about you and the cancer are described in this chapter and listed in **Guide 3.**

Health history

Expect your team to review your health in detail. This is known as taking a medical history. Your team will want to know a lot about your past and current health:

- Illnesses and injuries
- Symptoms like unexplained weight loss, trouble breathing, chest pain, and cough
- Prescribed and over-the-counter medicines and supplements
- Previous surgeries
- Lifestyle choices, including your diet, how active you are, and whether you smoke or drink alcohol

Some cancers and other diseases run in families. Be prepared to discuss the health of your close blood relatives. Such family members include siblings, parents, and grandparents related to you by birth.

Physical exam

A team member will also perform a thorough physical exam of your body. This exam may include:

- Checking your vital signs—blood pressure, heart rate, breathing rate, and body temperature
- Feeling or listening to organs, including your lungs, spleen, and liver
- Feeling for enlarged lymph nodes, which are small disease-fighting structures throughout your body
- Assessing your level of pain, if any, when you are touched

Performance status

Performance status is your ability to do day-to-day activities. It is based on your health history and exam. Your team will use your performance status to decide if your body can endure intense treatment.

Blood tests

Blood tests are commonly used to screen for disease. They are also used to assess if cancer is affecting organs. Samples of your blood will be needed for these 2 blood tests:

- A complete blood count measures parts of the blood including counts of white blood cells, red blood cells, and platelets.
- A chemistry profile assesses sugar and natural salts in your body and how well your liver and kidneys are working.

Lung cancer stages

Testing is needed to stage lung cancer. There are 4 main stages. You may see them written with Roman numerals:

Stage I (1)

Stage II (2)

Stage III (3)

Stage IV (4)

More information on cancer stages is in *Chapter 5: Planning primary treatment*.

Guide 3 First tests for early and locally advanced non-small cell lung cancer
• Medical history including weight loss and smoking history
• Physical exam
• Performance status
• Complete blood count
• Chemistry profile
• Diagnostic CT scan of the chest and upper abdomen with contrast

CT scan

Diagnostic computed tomography (CT) is often the first scan done to stage lung cancer.

A CT scan is a more detailed kind of x-ray. It takes many pictures from different angles. A computer combines the images to make 3D pictures.

You'll receive an injection of contrast if it's safe for you. Contrast is a substance that makes images clearer.

Your team will look for tumors in your chest and upper abdomen, including the adrenal glands. You'll need more CT scans if your current scans were done more than 60 days ago. Old scans should not be used to plan treatment.

Tests before treatment

Using the first set of tests, your team will start deciding what the stage of the cancer is. You may have more tests to confirm the stage and your treatment options. A list of possible additional tests is in **Guide 4.**

Imaging

Other types of imaging may be done to further assess where the lung cancer may have spread.

FDG-PET/CT scan
If not done before, positron emission tomography (PET) combined with a CT scan is necessary. PET/CT scans taken more than 60 days before should not be used to decide your treatment.

Your whole body will be scanned, or the scan will extend from your neck to the middle of your thighs. Before the scan, you will be injected with a radiotracer called fluorodeoxyglucose (FDG). The tracer makes even small amounts of cancer cells show up as hot (or bright) spots on the scan.

Brain MRI
Lung cancer tends to spread to the brain. Most people with lung cancer need a brain scan, but a brain scan isn't always needed for early cancers.

Magnetic resonance imaging (MRI) may show small brain tumors that aren't causing symptoms. MRI uses a safe magnetic field and radio waves to make images. Contrast will also be used unless it is not safe for you. If you can't have an MRI, you may get a CT scan of your head with contrast.

MRI of spine and thoracic inlet
Superior sulcus tumors are lung cancers that start at the top of the lung. They typically grow into the chest wall and may grow next to your spine, blood vessels, or nerves. If these tumors have grown through the chest wall, MRI of your spine and thoracic inlet is needed. The thoracic inlet is the center of a ring of bones at the top of the ribcage.

Pulmonary function tests

Pulmonary function tests are breathing activities used to assess how well your lungs work. Your team will use the results to decide if certain treatments are safe.

Bronchoscopy

A bronchoscopy is a procedure that allows your team to see inside your airways. It is done with a medical device called a bronchoscope. A bronchoscope has a small, flexible tube that is gently guided down your throat and into your airways.

A bronchoscopy is needed if:

- You haven't already had a bronchoscopy for diagnosis or cancer staging, and
- The lung cancer will be treated with surgery.

A bronchoscopy is often done on the day of surgery to save time, costs, and risks. Sometimes, a bronchoscopy is done before surgery for a tumor in the middle of a lung.

Lymph node biopsy

When lung cancer spreads, it typically spreads to lymph nodes in the lung and then to lymph nodes outside the lung. Your care team will use imaging to decide which, if any, lymph nodes to sample for cancer testing. Biopsy results are used to assess the cancer stage.

Mediastinal lymph nodes

The space between your lungs, called the mediastinum, has many lymph nodes. Lung cancer is more likely to spread to these nodes when the tumor is larger and closer to this area.

Mediastinal lymph nodes can be reached by one of several procedures:

- Mediastinoscopy is performed using a medical device that is inserted through a small cut in the chest.
- Mediastinotomy is an open surgery of the middle of the chest done through a small cut near the breastbone.
- Endoscopic ultrasound (EUS)-guided biopsy is performed using a medical device that is guided down your body's food tube (esophagus).
- Endobronchial ultrasound (EBUS)-guided biopsy is performed using a bronchoscope.

Guide 4
Possible tests for early and locally advanced non-small cell lung cancer

Imaging	• FDG-PET/CT scan • Brain MRI • MRI of spine and thoracic inlet
Lung tests	• Pulmonary function tests • Bronchoscopy
Cancer cell tests	• Lymph node biopsy • Biomarker tests

EBUS- and EUS-guided lymph node biopsies are often done days ahead of surgical treatment.

Other regional lymph nodes

Some lung cancers have spread to lymph nodes in the other lung or near the collarbone. Methods to biopsy these nodes include:

- An excisional biopsy removes an entire node through a cut into the skin.
- Thoracoscopy is a surgery that makes small openings into your chest through which small tools are inserted to see and remove tissue (also called video-assisted thoracoscopic surgery, or VATS).
- An external needle biopsy involves guiding a thin needle through your skin and into a node.

Biomarker tests

Biomarker tests look for biological clues, or markers, that experts use to make care decisions. Biomarkers differ between cancers and people.

Not everyone with early and locally advanced NSCLC needs biomarker testing. Biomarker testing may be done if you will receive drug treatment. Your team will plan treatment based on which biomarkers your cancer has.

Biomarker tests are performed on tumor tissue removed during a biopsy or surgery. A blood sample also may be tested.

PD-L1 level

PD-L1 is a protein on the surface of cells. PD-L1 on cancer cells stops white blood cells called T cells from killing cancer cells. The cancer cells then survive and make more cancer cells.

Lymph node biopsy

It is very important for your care team to know which lymph nodes have cancer. There are a few methods for examining or removing lymph nodes in the lungs and between the lungs. Bronchoscopy is one of those methods.

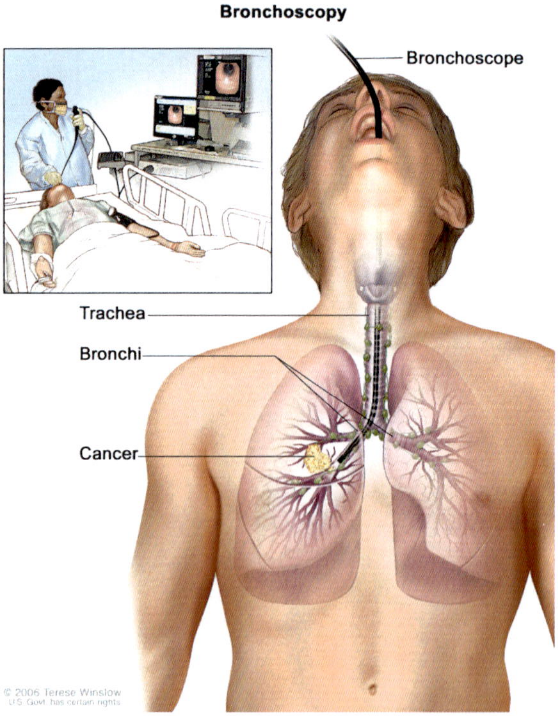

NCCN experts recommend PD-L1 testing to assess options for drug treatment.

EGFR mutations

Lung cancer cells have receptors on their surface called EGFR. Cell receptors receive and send signals like antennas.

Some mutations in the gene that makes EGFR cause the receptor to be overactive. EGFR overactivity makes the cancer cells quickly grow. Among *EGFR* mutations, *EGFR* exon 19 deletion and *EGFR* exon 21 *L858R* mutation are the most common.

Testing for *EGFR* mutations is needed to plan drug treatment used with surgery and drug treatment that follows chemoradiation.

ALK gene rearrangement

Some lung cancer cells grow quickly due to an overactive ALK surface receptor. The overactivity is caused when parts of two genes switch places with each other. This is called a gene rearrangement.

Testing for an *ALK* gene rearrangement is needed to plan drug treatment used with surgery.

What's next?

Your team will explain the test results to you and what they recommend for your cancer care.

A care plan usually includes treatment for cancer and support for you. NCCN experts recommend starting supportive care early. You'll find more information in *Chapter 4: Improving life with supportive care.*

To learn what NCCN experts recommend for the main treatment of lung cancer, read *Chapter 5: Planning primary treatment.*

Key points

- Your care team will make a treatment plan based on your test results and wishes.
- A member of your team will ask about your health, examine your body, and test blood samples.
- Imaging can help show where the cancer may have spread.
- Your ability to breathe may be tested with pulmonary function tests, and your lungs may be examined by bronchoscopy.
- To help stage the cancer, samples of lymph nodes inside or outside the lungs may be removed and tested for cancer.
- Biomarker tests look for small yet important features of cancer that differ between people. There are treatments for some biomarkers.

Questions to ask

- Could the tests be wrong or cause health problems?
- Will I need to pay any costs for the tests?
- What are the procedures for removing and storing tissue samples for future testing?
- How can I get a copy of the test results in case I want a second opinion?
- What do I need to do to prepare for testing?

4

Improving life with supportive care

28 What is supportive care?

28 Start supportive care early

28 Help to quit smoking

29 Managing common cancer effects

30 Addressing social and financial needs

30 What's next?

31 Key points

31 Questions to ask

Supportive care aims to improve your quality of life. A key part of care is reducing symptoms caused by cancer or treatment. Supportive care also provides help for social and financial needs.

What is supportive care?

Supportive care helps improve your quality of life during and after cancer treatment. The goal is to prevent or manage side effects and symptoms, like pain and cancer-related fatigue. It also addresses the mental, social, and spiritual concerns faced by those with cancer.

Supportive care is available to everyone with cancer and their families, not just those at the end of life. Palliative care is another name for supportive care.

Supportive care can also help with:

- Making treatment decisions
- Coordinating your care
- Paying for care
- Planning for advance care and end of life

Start supportive care early

NCCN experts recommend combining supportive care with cancer care shortly after diagnosis of non-small cell lung cancer (NSCLC). Receiving supportive care early can be more helpful than starting supportive care later.

Specialists who may provide supportive care to you include a:

- Palliative care specialist
- Respiratory therapist
- Rehabilitation specialist
- Registered dietitian
- Social worker

Help to quit smoking

Smoking can limit how well cancer treatment works.

- If you don't smoke, it's important that you don't start now.
- If you do smoke, it is important to quit. It's never too late.

Nicotine addiction is one of the hardest addictions to stop. The stress of having cancer may make it harder to quit.

The NCCN Guidelines for Patients: Quitting Smoking provides critical support and guidance for people with cancer. This book explains how to best use the tools that exist to help you quit for good.

If you tried to quit before, try again. Most people slip or relapse before quitting for good.

Managing common cancer effects

People with different types of cancer experience common health issues. Cancers share some common symptoms because they disrupt the body in similar ways. Treatment is similar for different cancers and causes common side effects.

Information on managing common effects can be found in the library of NCCN Guidelines for Patients. Books from the supportive care series are briefly described next so that you can find the information you need.

Palliative care

The NCCN Guidelines for Patients: Palliative Care describes care for physical and emotional symptoms:

- Diarrhea, constipation, sleep issues
- Stress and grief

It also provides guidance on talking with your team about cancer treatment.

Distress

Everyone with cancer feels distressed at some point. It is normal to feel worried, sad, helpless, or angry. NCCN Guidelines for Patients: Distress During Cancer Care empowers people to get help for distress.

Supportive care resources

More information on supportive care is available at NCCN.org/patientguidelines and on the NCCN Patient Guides for Cancer app.

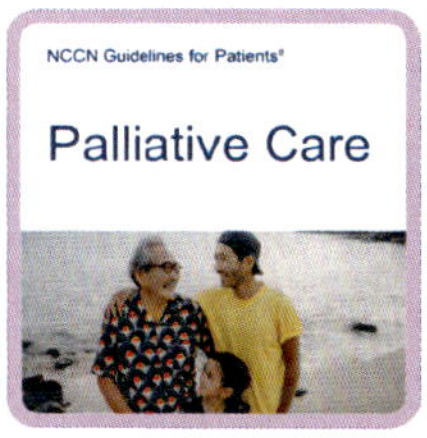

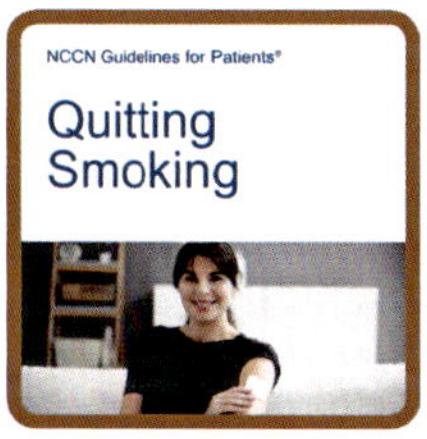

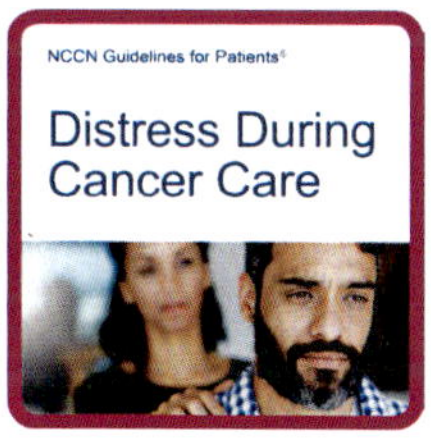

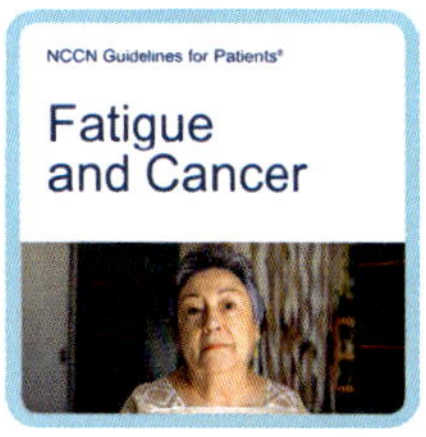

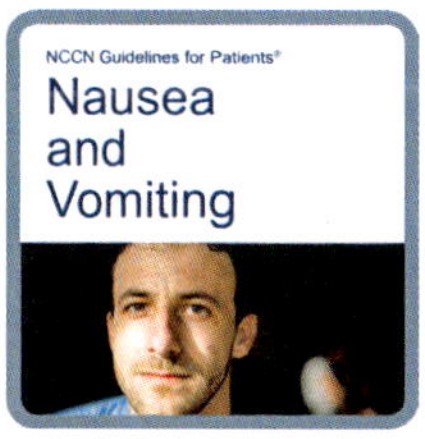

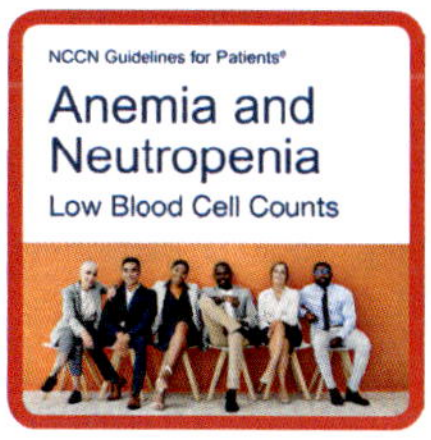

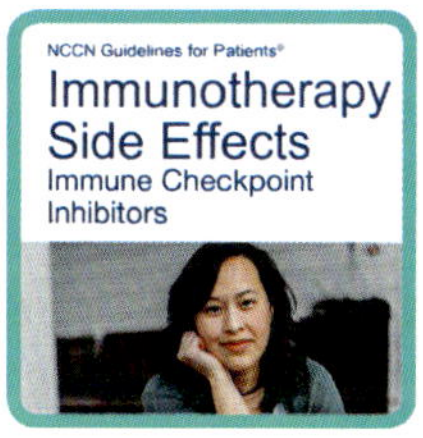

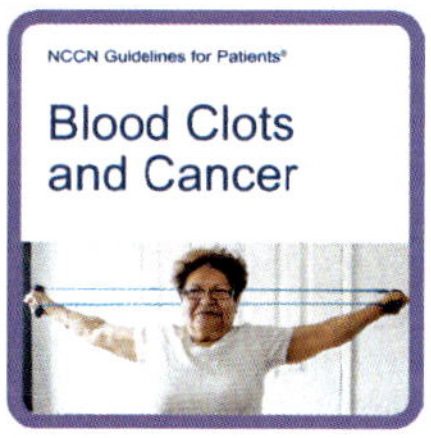

Fatigue

Cancer-related fatigue is not the typical tiredness that follows an active or long day. It's a lack of energy that is distressing, does not improve with normal rest or sleep, and disrupts life. Read the NCCN book on fatigue to learn about physical activity and other methods that reduce cancer-related fatigue.

Nausea and vomiting

Both chemotherapy and radiation therapy can cause nausea and vomiting. Nausea is the feeling that you are going to throw up. Vomiting is forcefully throwing up what's in your stomach. Treatments that prevent and manage both conditions are discussed in NCCN Guidelines for Patients: Nausea and Vomiting.

Anemia and neutropenia

Chemotherapy often causes a drop in red and white blood cells. A low number of red blood cells, called anemia, may cause fatigue. A low white blood cell count, called neutropenia, raises your risk of infections. Treatment for low blood cells is described in NCCN Guidelines for Patients: Anemia and Neutropenia.

Immunotherapy side effects

Immune checkpoint inhibitors are used to treat many types of NSCLC. This treatment may cause your immune cells to attack your healthy cells. NCCN Guidelines for Patients: Immunotherapy Side Effects: Immune Checkpoint Inhibitors explains treatment for:

- Skin and mouth symptoms
- Bowel and liver symptoms
- Thyroid, pituitary, and pancreas symptoms
- Lung symptoms

Blood clots

Some drug treatments for NSCLC increase the risk for blood clots. A thrombus is a type of blood clot that can dangerously block blood flow. The NCCN book on blood clots explains ways to prevent and treat thrombi.

Addressing social and financial needs

Many factors impact health outcomes. Your genes and health care are examples of important medical factors. But social factors are just as important. Social factors include:

- Transportation
- Housing and utility assistance
- Access to food
- Finances and work
- Health insurance
- Social support and safety

NCCN experts recommend that your team monitors the impact of social factors on your health. Your team will make referrals to other professionals as needed.

What's next?

Survivorship care is related to supportive care but focuses more on the long-term and late effects of cancer.

Although survivorship care often begins after initial treatment ends, many care recommendations can be started during treatment to prevent or lessen cancer-related effects.

To learn more, read *Chapter 9: Survivorship care.*

If you're looking for information on cancer treatment, a good place to start is *Chapter 5: Planning primary treatment.*

Key points

- Supportive care aims to improve your quality of life, including preventing and relieving symptoms.
- Starting supportive care early has more benefits than starting later.
- Quitting smoking may improve treatment results.

Questions to ask

- Should I tell health care providers I'm getting supportive care? They may incorrectly think I'm getting hospice care.
- What are the best methods to help me quit smoking?
- How will you prevent symptoms and relieve the symptoms I have?
- Who can assist me with getting help for social and financial needs?
- Who should I contact if my symptoms get worse?

5

Planning primary treatment

33 Types of primary treatment

34 Cancer staging with the TNM system

36 Treatment options by clinical stage

38 A clinical trial may be an option

40 What's next?

40 Key points

40 Questions to ask

Primary treatment is the main treatment used to rid your body of lung cancer. The options for primary treatment depend a lot on the cancer stage. Read this chapter to learn what your options for primary treatment may be.

Types of primary treatment

Treatment of early or locally advanced non-small cell lung cancer (NSCLC) may consist of one treatment or multiple types of treatments.

The treatment that is most important is called primary treatment. It either removes the cancer or kills the cancer cells.

Not everyone with NSCLC has the same primary treatment. The best treatment for you may not be the best treatment for someone else.

The 3 main types of primary treatment for early and locally advanced NSCLC are:

- **Surgery** is a treatment that removes tumors or organs with cancer. When possible, surgery is used for primary treatment of NSCLC. For many people, other types of treatments are received before or after surgery.
- **Radiation therapy** most often uses high-energy x-rays to treat lung cancer. When the goal is to cure cancer, it is called definitive radiation therapy.
- **Chemoradiation** uses both cancer drugs and radiation therapy to treat cancer. When the goal is to cure cancer, chemoradiation is called definitive chemoradiation.

Your care team will recommend a primary treatment for you. Which primary treatment you receive will depend largely on the cancer stage. A cancer stage is a rating of the growth and spread of cancer.

Read on to learn how lung cancer is staged and the treatment options for each stage.

> “Keep seeking out information and read information again as the diagnosis and treatment process continues."

Cancer staging with the TNM system

Your care team will stage the lung cancer using the tumor, node, metastasis (TNM) system maintained by the American Joint Committee on Cancer. Each letter in the system represents an area of cancer growth and will be assigned a score.

T = Tumor score

The T score describes the primary tumor. The primary tumor is the main group of cancer cells in the lung. The T scores are based on:

- The size of the primary tumor measured in centimeters (cm)
- Invasive growth of the primary tumor into nearby body parts, such as the chest wall
- The number of tumors in a lung

A brief description of T scores used in this book is in **Guide 5.**

Guide 5
T scores used to stage lung cancer

T1	A T1 tumor is 3 cm or smaller. It's no larger than a grape.
T2a	A T2a tumor is larger than 3 cm but no larger than 4 cm. It may have grown into the inner lining of the lung or the main airway. It may have caused the lung to collapse or swell.
T2b	A T2b tumor is larger than 4 cm but no larger than 5 cm. For comparison, a golf ball is 4.3 cm. The lung tumor may have grown into the inner lining of the lung or the main airway. It may have caused the lung to collapse or inflame.
T3	A T3 tumor may have one or more of these features: • Tumor size is larger than 5 cm but no larger than 7 cm • Invasive growth into the chest wall, phrenic nerve, outer lining of the lung, or heart's lining • Multiple related tumors in same lobe of the lung
T4	A T4 tumor may have one or more of these features: • Tumor size is larger than 7 cm • Invasive growth into the diaphragm, middle of the chest, heart, or its major blood vessels; windpipe or the area below; nerve to the voice box, esophagus, or spine • Related tumors in more than one lobe of the lung

N = Node score

The N score describes cancer growth in nearby lymph nodes. Lymph nodes are small, oval-shaped structures that are throughout your body and help fight disease. The N score is based on the spread of lung cancer to:

- Lymph nodes in the lung
- Lymph nodes just outside the lung
- Lymph nodes far from the lung

A brief description of N scores used in this book is in **Guide 6.**

M = Metastasis score

The M score tells you if the cancer has spread to the lining around the lung or to other organs. The spread of cancer is called metastasis.

Lung cancer tends to travel to the brain, liver, adrenal glands, and bones and from one lung to the other.

M0 means the cancer has not spread far. M1 means the cancer has spread far. There are three M1 scores to describe where the cancer has spread:

- M1a means the cancer has spread far within the chest.
- M1b means the cancer has spread to one place beyond the chest.
- M1c means the cancer has spread to more than one place beyond the chest.

Guide 6
N scores used to stage lung cancer

N0	The cancer has not spread to lymph nodes.
N1	The cancer has spread to lymph nodes in the lung.
N2	The cancer has spread to lymph nodes in one or both of these places: • In the middle of the chest next to the lung with cancer • Below the windpipe
N3	The cancer has spread to lymph nodes in one or more of these places: • In the middle of the chest near the other lung • In the other lung • Near the collarbone

Staging based on TNM scores

The stage of your cancer is determined by the TNM scores. TNM scores with a better outlook have a lower cancer stage.

TNM scores and the corresponding cancer stage are listed in **Guide 7.**

Guide 7
Stages of lung cancer

Cancer stage	TNM score
1A	T1, N0, M0
1B	T2a, N0, M0
2A	T2b, N0, M0
2B	T3, N0, M0 T1, N1, M0 T2, N1, M0
3A	T3, N1, M0 T4, N0, M0 T4, N1, M0 T1, N2, M0 T2, N2, M0
3B	T3, N2, M0 T4, N2, M0 T1, N3, M0 T2, N3, M0
3C	T3, N3, M0 T4, N3, M0
4A	Any T, Any N, M1a Any T, Any N, M1b
4B	Any T, Any N, M1c

There are 4 main stages of lung cancer. The cancer stages are further divided into subgroups and labeled with a letter.

- Stage 1 consists of stage 1A and 1B
- Stage 2 consists of stage 2A and 2B
- Stage 3 consists of stage 3A, 3B, and 3C
- Stage 4 consists of stage 4A and 4B

All lung cancers are staged before treatment based on the tests described in *Chapter 3: Testing for early and locally advanced NSCLC*. The pretreatment stage is called the clinical stage.

If you have surgery, the cancer is staged again. The second stage is called the pathologic stage. It is based on tests of tissue removed from your body.

Treatment options by clinical stage

The clinical stage is very important for planning primary treatment. It helps predict the course of the cancer and which treatment is best.

Options for primary treatment of early and locally advanced NSCLC vary based on the T and N scores:

- The size, number, and location of lung tumors affect treatment options.
- Options also differ for lung tumors that have grown through the wall of the lung and into other tissue. This is called invasive growth.

- Also important is which lymph nodes, if any, have cancer.

Options for primary treatment by clinical stage are noted in **Guide 8.**

Your team will make a final recommendation for treatment based on additional factors. These factors include any challenges to treatment, your lung functioning, and your overall health. Your team's recommendation will also reflect your values and preferences.

Guide 8
Options for primary treatment of early and locally advanced NSCLC

Clinical stage	TNM score	Surgery	Definitive radiation therapy	Definitive chemoradiation
1A	T1, N0, M0	●	●	
1B	T2a, N0, M0	●	●	
2A	T2b, N0, M0	●	●	
2B	T3 (no invasive growth), N0, M0	●	●	
2B	T3 (invasive growth), N0, M0 T1, N1, M0 T2, N1, M0	●		●
3A	T3, N1, M0 T4, N0, M0 T4, N1, M0 T1, N2, M0 T2, N2, M0	●		●
3B	T3, N2, M0	●		●
3B	T4, N2, M0 T1, N3, M0 T2, N3, M0			●
3C	T3, N3, M0 T4, N3, M0			●

A clinical trial may be an option

You may be able to receive cancer treatment in a clinical trial. A clinical trial is a type of medical research study. After being developed and tested in a lab, potential new ways of fighting cancer need to be studied in people.

If found to be safe and effective in a clinical trial, a drug, device, or treatment approach may be approved by the U.S. Food and Drug Administration (FDA).

Everyone with cancer should carefully consider all of the treatment options available for their cancer type, including standard treatments and clinical trials. Talk to your doctor about whether a clinical trial may make sense for you.

Phases

Most cancer clinical trials focus on treatment and are done in phases.

- **Phase 1** trials study the safety and side effects of an investigational drug or treatment approach.
- **Phase 2** trials study how well the drug or approach works against a specific type of cancer.
- **Phase 3** trials test the drug or approach against a standard treatment. If the results are good, it may be approved by the FDA.
- **Phase 4** trials study the safety and benefit of an FDA-approved treatment.

"When you are deciding your treatment, remember that even though some decisions need to be made fast, don't rush. Think through your options and get second, or even third opinions. Have people you can trust to talk through your options so you feel comfortable in your decisions."

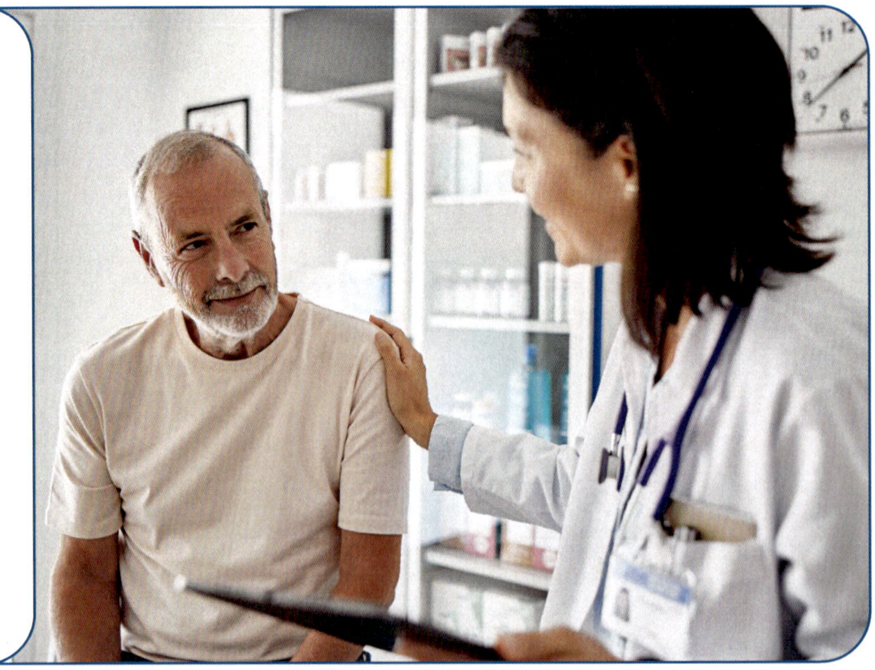

Who can enroll?

It depends on the clinical trial's rules, called eligibility criteria. The rules may be about age, cancer type and stage, treatment history, or general health. They ensure that participants are alike in specific ways and that the trial is as safe as possible for the participants.

Informed consent

Clinical trials are managed by a research team. This group of experts will review the study with you in detail, including its purpose and the risks and benefits of joining. All of this information is also provided in an informed consent form. Read the form carefully and ask questions before signing it. Take time to discuss it with people you trust. Keep in mind that you can leave and seek treatment outside of the clinical trial at any time.

Will I get a placebo?

Placebos (inactive versions of real medicines) are almost never used alone in cancer clinical trials. It is common to receive either a placebo with a standard treatment, or a new drug with a standard treatment. You will be informed, verbally and in writing, if a placebo is part of a clinical trial before you enroll.

Are clinical trials free?

There is no fee to enroll in a clinical trial. The study sponsor pays for research-related costs, including the study drug. But you may need to pay for other services, like transportation or childcare, due to extra appointments. During the trial, you will continue to receive standard cancer care. This care is often covered by insurance.

Finding a clinical trial

In the United States

NCCN Cancer Centers
NCCN.org/cancercenters

The National Cancer Institute (NCI)
cancer.gov/about-cancer/treatment/clinical-trials/search

Worldwide

The U.S. National Library of Medicine (NLM)
clinicaltrials.gov/

Need help finding a clinical trial?

NCI's Cancer Information Service (CIS)
1.800.4.CANCER (1.800.422.6237)
cancer.gov/contact

What's next?

Now that you know your options for primary treatment, you can find more information about your treatment in the next chapters.

- People who have surgery usually receive treatment in multiple phases because more than one type of treatment is used. Surgical procedures and treatments used with surgery are explained in *Chapter 6: Lung cancer surgery.*
- The types of radiation therapy that are used to cure lung cancer are described in *Chapter 7: Radiation therapy.*
- Options for chemotherapy that is given with radiation therapy are listed in *Chapter 8: Chemoradiation.*

Key points

- The 3 main treatments of early and locally advanced non-small cell lung cancer (NSCLC) are surgery, radiation therapy, and chemoradiation.
- Your options for treatment are based on a rating of the growth and spread of the cancer before treatment. This rating is called the clinical stage. There are 4 stages.
- Surgery is a standard treatment for stage 1, stage 2, and stage 3 NSCLC. If surgery is not an option, radiation therapy or chemoradiation may be used for treatment instead.
- Another possible option is a clinical trial. A clinical trial tests new ways of stopping cancer in people.

Questions to ask

- What is the clinical stage of the cancer?
- How did you decide what primary therapy I can have?
- Is there a clinical trial that's a good fit for me?

6
Lung cancer surgery

42 Planning treatment
44 Treatment before surgery
46 How lung cancer is removed
49 Treatment after surgery
50 Additional therapy after chemotherapy
51 What's next?
51 Key points
52 Questions to ask

Surgery is a standard treatment for lung cancer, but the treatment approach differs between people. Read this chapter to learn about the treatment you may have.

Planning treatment

Surgery, by itself or with other treatments, is used to treat most early-stage and many locally advanced non-small cell lung cancers (NSCLC). The goal of surgical treatment is to cure the cancer.

Evaluation for surgery

NCCN experts recommend finding a highly experienced, board-certified thoracic surgeon. Lung cancer surgery should be a major part of their practice.

Surgery may be an option for you if all the cancer can be safely removed. To decide if you can safely undergo surgery, your surgeon will consider:

- Where the cancer is in your lung and outside your lung
- The health of your lungs
- Your overall health

Cancer that can be safely and completely removed is called resectable cancer.

Evaluation for perioperative therapy

Resectable NSCLC is sometimes treated with more than one type of treatment. These other treatments may be received before or after surgery and are referred to as perioperative therapy.

Your care team will plan treatment based on several factors, including:

- The type and stage of NSCLC
- Your health history, including medicines you take
- Biomarker tests for PD-L1 level, *ALK* rearrangement, and *EGFR* mutations

Other types of treatments used with surgery are systemic therapy, radiation therapy, and chemoradiation.

Systemic therapy

Systemic therapy is commonly used for perioperative therapy. It is a whole-body treatment with cancer drugs. Types of systemic therapy are described in **Guide 9.**

A medical oncologist prescribes drug regimens to treat cancer. A regimen consists of one or more drugs that are taken at a specific dose, schedule, and length of time.

Radiation therapy

Radiation therapy is sometimes given after surgery. It treats cancer that may remain near the surgical site.

The specialist who plans radiation therapy is called a radiation oncologist. Details about receiving radiation therapy are in *Chapter 7: Radiation therapy.*

Chemoradiation

Chemoradiation is treatment with both chemotherapy and radiation therapy.

- Sequential chemoradiation is the use of one treatment and then the other.
- Concurrent chemoradiation is the use of both treatments during the same time frame.

More information is in *Chapter 8: Chemoradiation.*

Side effects of treatment

Side effects are unwanted health issues caused by treatment.

All cancer treatments cause side effects. Side effects vary between people based on the type and length of treatment as well as differences among people.

Management of side effects is discussed in *Chapter 4: Supportive care*.

Guide 9
Systemic therapies used before or after surgery for NSCLC

Platinum-doublet chemotherapy	• Chemotherapy kills fast-growing cells including cancer cells. • Platinum-doublet chemotherapy consists of either cisplatin or carboplatin and a second drug. The second drug is either pemetrexed (Alimta, Pemfexy), paclitaxel, vinorelbine, etoposide (Toposar, Etopophos), gemcitabine (Gemzar, Infugem), or docetaxel (Docivyx,Taxotere). • Chemotherapy is given by a slow drip into a vein, called an infusion, and occurs in cycles of treatment days followed by days of rest.
Immune checkpoint inhibitors	• Immune checkpoint inhibitors restore the ability of immune T cells to kill cancer cells. • Atezolizumab (Tecentriq), pembrolizumab (Keytruda), durvalumab (Imfinzi), and nivolumab (Opdivo) are immune checkpoint inhibitors. They are given by infusion in cycles. • Atezolizumab with hyaluronidase-tqjs (Tecentriq Hybreza) and nivolumab with hyaluronidase-nvhy (Opdivo Qvantig) are injections under the skin.
Targeted therapy	• Alectinib (Alecensa) and osimertinib (Tagrisso) are targeted therapies that stop chemical signals that tell lung cancer cells to grow. • Both are pills that can be taken at home on treatment days of the cycle.

Treatment before surgery

Preoperative therapy is treatment that is received before surgery. It is sometimes called neoadjuvant therapy or induction therapy.

The clinical stage of the cancer is an important factor when planning preoperative therapy. For example, NCCN experts don't recommend preoperative therapy for stage 1 cancers because surgery alone has very good results.

Preoperative instead of postoperative therapy

For years, systemic therapy occurred after surgery for many stage 2 and 3A cancers. Treatment after surgery is called postoperative therapy.

More recently, these cancers have been treated with preoperative therapy instead. Preoperative therapy prolongs life just like postoperative therapy but can have less serious side effects.

NCCN experts recommend that care teams evaluate for preoperative therapy when the lung tumor is at least 4 centimeters (cm) in size or the cancer has spread to lymph nodes.

If your team recommends preoperative therapy, you will receive:

- An **immune checkpoint inhibitor and chemotherapy** from **Guide 10.**
- If immune checkpoint inhibitors aren't an option, **platinum-doublet chemotherapy** from **Guide 11.**

Guide 10
Immune checkpoint inhibitors and chemotherapy by types of NSCLC

Adenocarcinoma, large cell carcinoma, and rare cell types

Regimens used with nivolumab or nivolumab and hyaluronidase-tqjs:

- Carboplatin, paclitaxel
- Cisplatin, pemetrexed
- Cisplatin, paclitaxel
- Carboplatin, pemetrexed

Regimen used with pembrolizumab:

- Cisplatin, pemetrexed

Regimens used with durvalumab:

- Cisplatin, pemetrexed
- Carboplatin, pemetrexed

Squamous cell carcinoma

Regimens used with nivolumab:

- Carboplatin, paclitaxel
- Cisplatin, gemcitabine
- Cisplatin, paclitaxel
- Carboplatin, gemcitabine

Regimen used with pembrolizumab:

- Cisplatin, gemcitabine

Regimens used with durvalumab:

- Carboplatin, paclitaxel
- Cisplatin, gemcitabine
- Carboplatin, gemcitabine

Regimens for platinum-doublet chemotherapy are grouped by NCCN levels of preference:

- **Preferred therapies** have the most evidence they work better and may be safer than other therapies.
- **Other recommended therapies** may not work quite as well as preferred therapies, but they can still help treat cancer.
- **Therapies used in certain cases** work best for people with specific cancer features or health circumstances.

You may have additional therapy after surgery. Options are discussed later in this chapter in the section called *Treatment after surgery.*

Shrinking cancer before surgery

For some lung cancers, preoperative therapy is given to shrink the cancer and make surgery easier.

Stage 2 and stage 3 invasive tumors

Invasive tumors have grown through the wall of the lung and into other tissues. Concurrent chemoradiation or systemic therapy may be received before surgery for:

- Stage 2B and stage 3A cancers with T3 tumors that invaded tissue near the lung
- Stage 3A cancers with T4 tumors

Stage 2 and stage 3 superior sulcus tumors

Concurrent chemoradiation is the first treatment of superior sulcus tumors. Superior sulcus tumors are a distinct subset of invasive lung cancers. They start at the top of the lung and typically grow into the chest wall.

Guide 11
Platinum-doublet chemotherapy by types of NSCLC

Adenocarcinoma, large cell carcinoma, and rare cell types

Preferred therapy:

- Cisplatin, pemetrexed

Other recommended therapies:

- Cisplatin, vinorelbine
- Cisplatin, etoposide

Therapies used in certain cases:

- Carboplatin, paclitaxel
- Carboplatin, pemetrexed

Squamous cell carcinoma

Preferred therapies:

- Cisplatin, gemcitabine
- Cisplatin, docetaxel

Other recommended therapies:

- Cisplatin, vinorelbine
- Cisplatin, etoposide

Therapies used in certain cases:

- Carboplatin, paclitaxel
- Carboplatin, gemcitabine

Not all of these cancers will be treated with surgery. If surgery isn't possible, chemoradiation becomes the main treatment and is finished with the goal of curing the cancer.

Stage 3 with cancer in N2 nodes

NSCLC with an N2 stage is sometimes treated with surgery. To make this possible, preoperative systemic therapy or preoperative chemoradiation is given first to stop cancer growth.

How lung cancer is removed

Your surgeon will schedule surgery if there's a good chance that all the cancer will be removed. They must see a way to remove the tumor with enough normal-looking tissue at its edge. This normal-looking tissue is called the surgical margin. The goal is to have no cancer cells in the margin so that a cure is likely.

Methods to perform surgery

Your surgeon will remove tissue with one of two methods. The classic or open method is called thoracotomy. The newer method is a less invasive surgery called thoracoscopy.

Thoracotomy is performed through one large cut between the ribs. Surgical tools are inserted through the cut to remove the cancer. Sometimes, part of the rib needs to be removed, too.

Thoracoscopy is performed through several small cuts between the ribs. This surgery is sometimes called video-assisted thoracoscopic surgery because it is performed using a small video camera inserted through a cut.

Your surgeon may perform thoracoscopy using robotic arms to control the surgical tools. This approach is called robotic-assisted thoracoscopic surgery.

Exploring inside the chest

During surgery, your surgeon will explore your inner chest to see where cancer is growing. Surgery allows for a better view of the tumor compared to imaging scans. Also, areas of growth that weren't seen on scans may be found during surgery.

Types of lung surgery

The type of surgery you will have depends on where the tumor has grown and how well your lungs work.

The right lung has 3 parts (lobes), and the left lung has 2 lobes. Some tumors are found in only in 1 lobe of the lung. Other tumors have grown from 1 lobe into another lobe or have grown outside the lung.

Your surgeon will perform one of these 5 surgeries based on where the tumor has grown:

- **Wedge resection** removes a small part of a lobe.
- **Segmentectomy** removes a large part of a lobe.
- **Lobectomy** removes an entire lobe and is preferred for most lung cancers.
- **Sleeve lobectomy** removes an entire lobe and part of the main airway.

- **Pneumonectomy** removes an entire lung.

Lung tumors that have grown through the lung wall into other tissue will be removed in one piece. This surgery is called an en-bloc resection.

Types of lymph node surgery

During surgery, your surgeon will also remove lymph nodes that have or may have cancer. To remove nodes, some organs may need to be moved or cut. There are 2 types of lymph node surgery:

- A systematic lymph node sampling removes some nodes in the lung and between the lungs.
- A lymph node dissection removes as many nodes as possible from the lung and between the lungs.

Lung cancer surgery

There are 5 common lung cancer surgeries. The most common are lobectomy and pneumonectomy and are shown below. A sleeve lobectomy removes a lobe and part of the main airway called the bronchus. Wedge resection and segmentectomy remove only part of a lobe.

Lobectomy

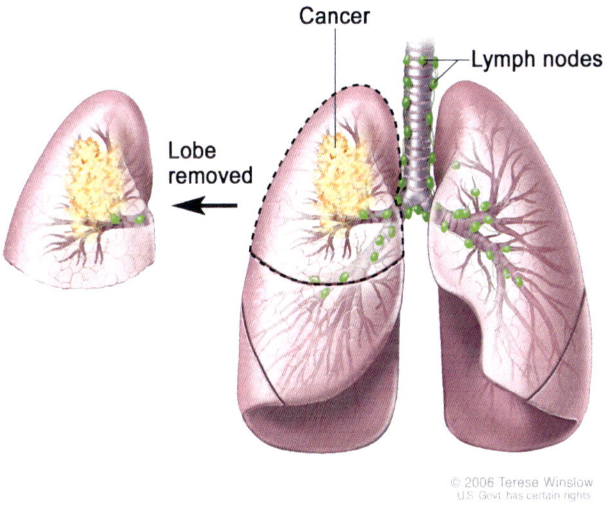

Pneumonectomy

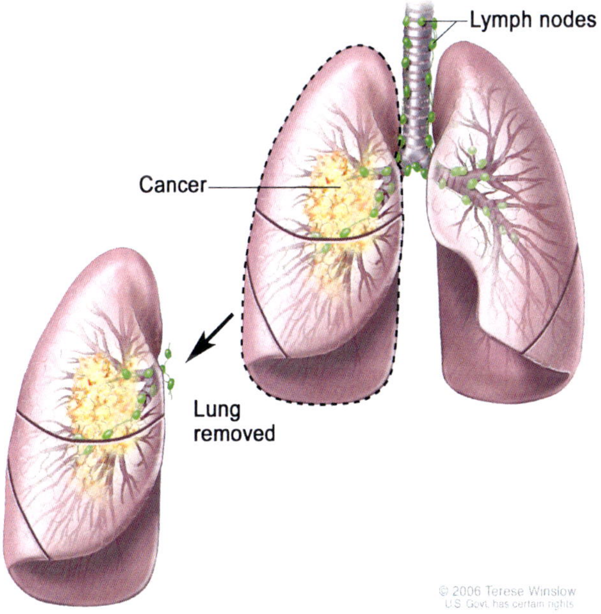

Looking for cancer in surgical tissue

After surgery, your surgeon and pathologist will rate the surgical margin around the removed tumor:

- **R0** means no cancer was found in the margin.
- **R1** means cancer was found in the margin with a microscope.
- **R2** means some of the visible cancer wasn't removed.

The pathologist will also assess fluid samples and removed lymph nodes for cancer. When lymph nodes farthest from the tumor don't have cancer, it is likely that all nodes with cancer were removed.

Surgery is described as a complete resection when surgical margins, the furthest lymph nodes, and the fluid around the lungs and heart are cancer-free.

Side effects of surgery

Your care team will help you recover from surgery. They will provide care to prevent or relieve side effects.

Common side effects of any surgery are pain, swelling, and scars. Pain can be intense after lung surgery. Pain and swelling often fade away in the weeks after surgery.

Surgical margin

The tumor will be removed, along with some normal-looking tissue around its rim. The normal-looking tissue is called the surgical margin. The surgical margin will be tested for cancer. Postoperative therapy is based on if there is cancer in the margins.

R0 margin
No cancer in margin

R1 margin
Cancer is found in margin with lab tests

R2 margin
Cancer is easily seen in margin

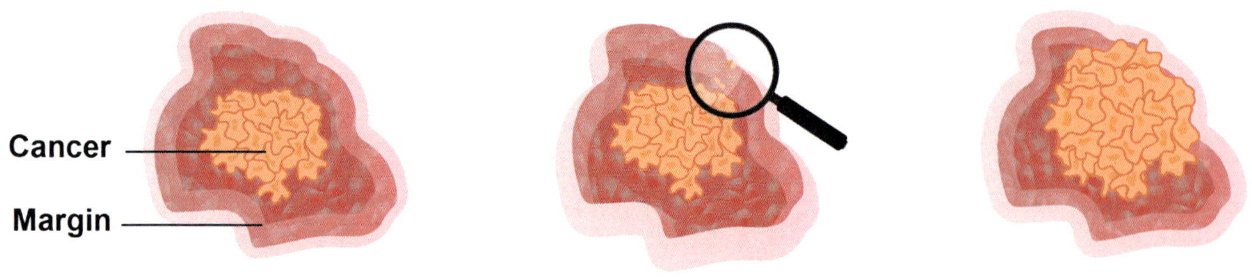

Treatment after surgery

After surgery, you may have postoperative therapy (also called adjuvant therapy). Postoperative therapy treats cancer that likely wasn't removed during surgery. It lowers the chance of cancer returning.

No cancer in surgical margins (R0)

You may receive postoperative therapy even if margins are cancer-free. Some cancer may remain in your body because it wasn't seen or detected with scans.

NCCN experts recommend postoperative chemotherapy for:

- Stage 1B cancers that are highly likely to return, including those 4 cm in size
- Stage 2A cancers that are highly likely to return
- Stage 2B cancers
- Stage 3 cancers

Regimens used for postoperative chemotherapy are the same as those used for preoperative therapy. Options are listed earlier in this chapter in **Guide 11.**

If postoperative chemotherapy is not an option, you may receive targeted therapy with osimertinib if the cancer has *EGFR* mutations.

Cancer in surgical margins (R1, R2)

Postoperative therapy is needed when cancer is in the surgical margins. It is very likely that the cancer was not fully removed.

Options to treat cancer that remains after surgery are a second surgery, radiation therapy, and chemoradiation

Second surgery

A second surgery to remove all the cancer is an option for stage 1 and stage 2 cancers. It is preferred over other options for stage 1 and stage 2A.

After the second surgery, NCCN experts recommend postoperative chemotherapy for:

- Stage 1B cancers that are highly likely to return, including those 4 cm in size
- Stage 2A cancers that are highly likely to return
- Stage 2B cancers

Radiation therapy

Radiation therapy is another way to treat any cancer that's still in your body. It's an option for stage 1 and stage 2A cancers when a second surgery is likely to cause serious health issues.

Chemoradiation

Stage 2A cancers with R2 margins are sometimes treated with chemoradiation instead of radiation therapy alone.

If you haven't had chemoradiation before, it is an option for stage 2B and stage 3 cancers.

- Either sequential or concurrent chemoradiation is recommended for R1 margins.
- Concurrent chemoradiation is recommended when there are R2 margins.

Regimens used for sequential chemoradiation are listed earlier in this chapter in **Guide 11.**

Regimens used with concurrent chemoradiation are listed in *Chapter 8: Chemoradiation.*

Additional therapy after chemotherapy

NCCN experts recommend that care teams assess the need for additional treatment when completely removed cancers were at least 4 cm in size or had spread to lymph nodes.

Due to their size or the spread to nodes, these cancers are more likely to return than other cancers. Additional treatment may lower the chance of them returning.

Cancers with ALK and or EGFR biomarkers

Cancers with *ALK* rearrangements or *EGFR* mutations may be treated with targeted therapy:

- Cancers with *ALK* rearrangements may be treated with alectinib.
- After postoperative chemotherapy, cancers with *EGFR* mutations may be treated with osimertinib.

Cancers without ALK or EGFR biomarkers

Cancers without *ALK* rearrangements or *EGFR* mutations may be treated with immune checkpoint inhibitors:

After preoperative chemotherapy

- If you had preoperative durvalumab and chemotherapy, durvalumab may be restarted.
- If you had preoperative nivolumab and chemotherapy, nivolumab may be restarted. Nivolumab with hyaluronidase-nvhy injections may be used instead of intravenous nivolumab.
- If you had preoperative pembrolizumab and chemotherapy, pembrolizumab may be restarted.

After postoperative chemotherapy

- Cancers with PD-L1 may be treated with atezolizumab. Atezolizumab and hyaluronidase-tqjs injections may be used instead of intravenous atezolizumab.
- After postoperative chemotherapy, cancers may be treated with pembrolizumab.

What's next?

Once there are no signs of cancer, you'll have ongoing testing to watch out for the return of cancer. This is called surveillance and it's a part of survivorship care.

Survivorship care also focuses on the management of long-term and late effects of cancer. To learn more, read *Chapter 9: Survivorship care.*

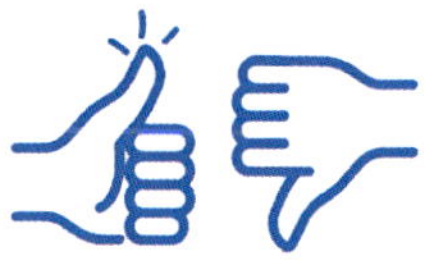

Let us know what you think!

Please take a moment to complete an online survey about the NCCN Guidelines for Patients.
NCCN.org/patients/response

Key points

- Choose a highly experienced, board-certified thoracic surgeon who can remove all the cancer safely.
- Depending on the cancer stage and other factors, you may have systemic therapy or chemoradiation before surgery.
- There are several types of lung surgery that range from removing a piece of a lobe to removing the entire lung. Lymph nodes that have or may have cancer are removed, too.
- Lung cancer surgery can be performed by one of two methods. During open surgery, body tissue is removed through one large cut. Less invasive surgery is performed through a few small cuts.
- Postoperative therapy helps stop the cancer from returning. The type of treatment you'll have depends on many factors, including if cancer is in the removed tissue at the edge of the tumor.
- Additional drug treatment is sometimes given after chemotherapy to stop high-risk cancers from returning. You may receive a different type of treatment or one of your prior treatments may be restarted.

Questions to ask

- How many lung cancer surgeries have you done in the past year?
- What type of surgery do I need?
- Will I have other treatments before or after surgery?
- If drug treatment is needed, how often do I get treated and when will treatment be done?
- What are the common and serious side effects of my treatments?

"

Take your journey one second at a time. Each path is different and we just don't know where ours will lead."

7
Radiation therapy

54 Uses of radiation therapy

55 Types of radiation therapy

55 Curing lung cancer with radiation

56 Side effects of radiation

56 What's next?

57 Key points

57 Questions to ask

Radiation therapy is a common treatment for lung cancer. It may be used by itself to treat lung cancer or it can be combined with other treatments. This chapter explains when radiation therapy is used and how it works.

Uses of radiation therapy

Radiation therapy uses high-energy x-rays or particles to treat lung cancer. The x-rays or particles damage cancer cells, which either die or stop making new cancer cells.

Radiation therapy is used in many ways to treat early and locally advanced non-small cell lung cancer (NSCLC):

- It is used as the main (also called primary) treatment of stage 1 and some stage 2 lung cancers. When the goal is to cure cancer, it is called definitive radiation therapy.
- It is used with surgery as described in *Chapter 6: Lung cancer surgery.*
- It is combined with chemotherapy as described in *Chapter 8: Chemoradiation.*

A radiation oncologist is an expert in treating cancer with radiation. Your doctor will lead a team that designs your treatment plan and provides treatment.

Radiation therapy

Radiation therapy is often delivered from a large machine. The x-rays or particles pass through skin and travel to the tumor. Healthy tissue is protected using modern types of treatment.

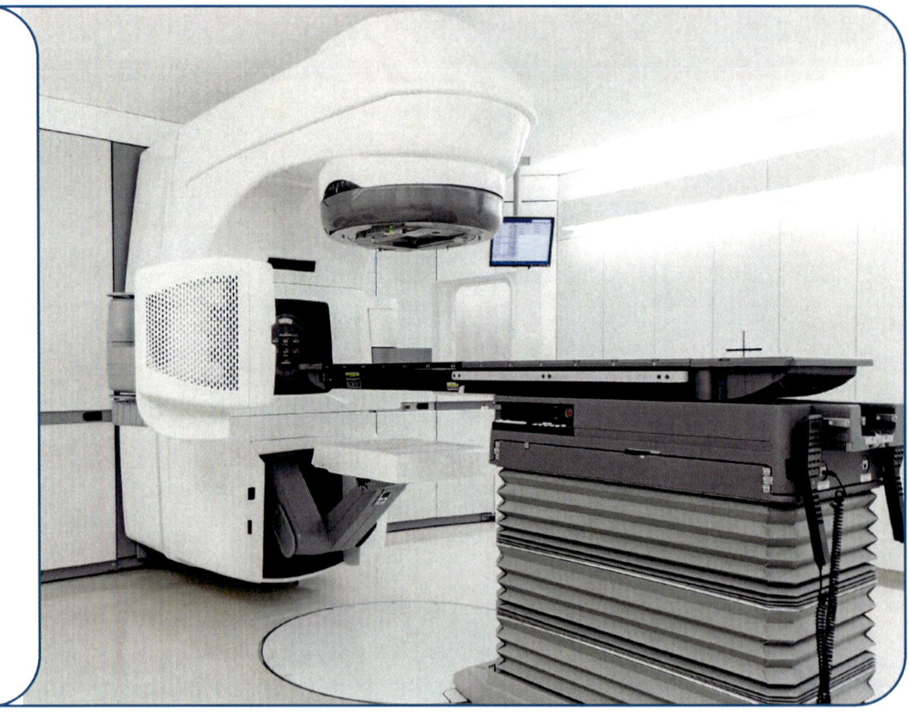

Types of radiation therapy

External beam radiation therapy (EBRT) is the most common method used for lung cancer. A large machine makes radiation beams that are shaped to the form of the tumor. The machine aims the highest radiation dose at the tumor. A much lower dose is given to the nearby normal-looking tissue.

There are several common techniques of EBRT:

- **Intensity-modulated radiation therapy (IMRT)** delivers x-ray (photon) beams that very closely match the shape of the target and spares more normal tissue.
- **Stereotactic ablative radiotherapy (SABR)** treats cancer with very precise, high-dose x-ray (photon) beams. It delivers a very high dose of radiation per treatment, so it's only given for a few treatments. Treatment is finished in 1 to 1½ weeks.
- **Proton therapy** treats cancer with proton beams. Proton beams deliver radiation mostly within the tumor.
- **Three-dimensional conformal radiation therapy (3D-CRT)** delivers an x-ray (photon) beam that matches the shape of the target but may not be as focused as IMRT. It is an older technique.

Radiation therapy is typically delivered daily from Monday through Friday. Treatment visits are about 15 minutes for IMRT and 3D-CRT and 30 to 45 minutes for SABR and proton therapy. Some radiation oncologists deliver SABR treatment 2 to 3 times per week.

Curing lung cancer with radiation

Definitive EBRT is used when trying to cure stage 1 and stage 2 NSCLC. Any of the EBRT techniques described may be used, though NCCN experts prefer SABR for smaller tumors. SABR may be an option for some stage 2 cancers with large T3 tumors.

Overcoming treatment challenges

A lung tumor is harder to target than some other tumors in the body. Lung tumors often move when you breathe. To account for these challenges, advanced methods may be used:

- Four-dimensional computed tomography (4D-CT) may be used for treatment planning. It's like a video, so your radiation oncologist will see how the tumor moves when you breathe.
- Motion control methods may be used to keep the tumor still during treatment.
- At times, your radiation oncologist may ask you to hold your breath for 15 to 20 seconds at a time to better target the tumor.

Adjuvant therapy

Adjuvant chemotherapy may be received after definitive radiation therapy. It treats cancer that radiation did not. For example, large tumors and very abnormal-looking cancer cells may have spread to places outside the radiation field.

Adjuvant chemotherapy is an option for stage 2 cancer that is highly likely to return. NCCN experts recommend that care teams especially consider chemotherapy for stage 2 cancers with T2b and T3 tumors.

See Guide 11 in Chapter 6 for a list of chemotherapy regimens used for adjuvant therapy.

Side effects of radiation

Radiation therapy does not cause pain during a treatment session—you'll feel nothing at all. It also does not make you radioactive. But radiation therapy may cause health issues called side effects.

Facts about side effects

Here are some important things to know:

- Side effects differ by the type of radiation therapy. Most people have no side effects from SABR. Proton therapy may cause skin changes, but IMRT rarely does.
- Side effects of radiation therapy are cumulative. This means they build up slowly and are worse at the end of treatment.
- Adding chemotherapy to radiation therapy often causes more side effects.
- Side effects that start during radiation therapy typically improve 2 to 4 weeks after treatment is finished.

Types of side effects

During treatment, your radiation oncologist will see you about once a week to assess for possible side effects. Side effects that you may have include:

- Fatigue is a common side effect of radiation therapy.
- Skin changes in the treatment area may occur. Often, people describe skin changes as like a sunburn. For people with darker skin, radiation can cause the skin to darken and be painful.
- Near the end of treatment, you may have pain when swallowing due to irritation to your esophagus.
- Although not common, your lung may become inflamed after treatment causing sudden shortness of breath or cough. These are symptoms of radiation pneumonitis. Call your radiation oncologist immediately if you have these symptoms.

Management of side effects is discussed in *Chapter 4: Improving life with supportive care.*

What's next?

Once there are no signs of cancer, you'll have ongoing testing to watch out for the return of cancer. This is called surveillance and it's a part of survivorship care.

Survivorship care also focuses on the management of long-term and late effects of cancer. To learn more, read *Chapter 9: Survivorship care.*

Key points

- Radiation therapy uses high-energy x-rays or particles to treat lung cancer.
- There are several ways radiation therapy is used to treat lung cancer. When used to cure cancer, it is called definitive radiation therapy.
- Radiation therapy is most often delivered from outside the body using a large machine.
- Several techniques are available to cure lung cancer, but stereotactic ablative radiotherapy (SABR) is preferred for smaller tumors.
- You may receive chemotherapy to treat any cancer that radiation therapy did not.
- Side effects from radiation build up over the course of treatment and typically improve 2 to 4 weeks after treatment is done.

Questions to ask

- Why is radiation therapy being used to treat my cancer?
- Explain how you chose the type of radiation therapy to use?
- Do I need chemotherapy after radiation therapy?
- How will you try to prevent side effects of radiation?
- What are the long-term side effects of cancer.

8 Chemoradiation

59 Uses of chemoradiation

59 Types of chemotherapy

60 Curing lung cancer with chemoradiation

60 Consolidation treatment

61 Treatment side effects

62 What's next?

62 Key points

62 Questions to ask

Chemoradiation uses the power of two different cancer treatments. It may be used to cure lung cancer. Read this chapter to learn about chemoradiation options.

Chemoradiation is sometimes received before or after surgery as described in *Chapter 6: Lung cancer surgery.*

Chemoradiation may also be the main (also called primary) treatment of locally advanced lung cancer when surgery is not an option. When the goal is to cure cancer, it is called definitive chemoradiation.

Uses of chemoradiation

Chemoradiation is a cancer treatment that combines chemotherapy and radiation therapy:

- **Chemotherapy** uses drugs that stop the process by which cells make more cells, so it affects fast-growing cells like cancer cells.
- **Radiation therapy** uses high-energy x-rays or particles to damage cancer cells. The cancer cells either die or can't make more cancer cells.

Types of chemotherapy

Doctors called medical oncologists prescribe chemotherapy. A chemotherapy regimen consists of one or more drugs that are taken at a specific dose, schedule, and length of time.

For non-small cell lung cancer (NSCLC), more than one type of chemotherapy is often received. Most commonly, cisplatin or carboplatin is used with another drug. This is called platinum-doublet chemotherapy.

Chemotherapy

Chemotherapy for lung cancer is a liquid that is injected into a vein. Some injections are done in the arm or hand while others are done though an implanted device called a port. An infusion is a slow drip controlled by a pump that may take hours.

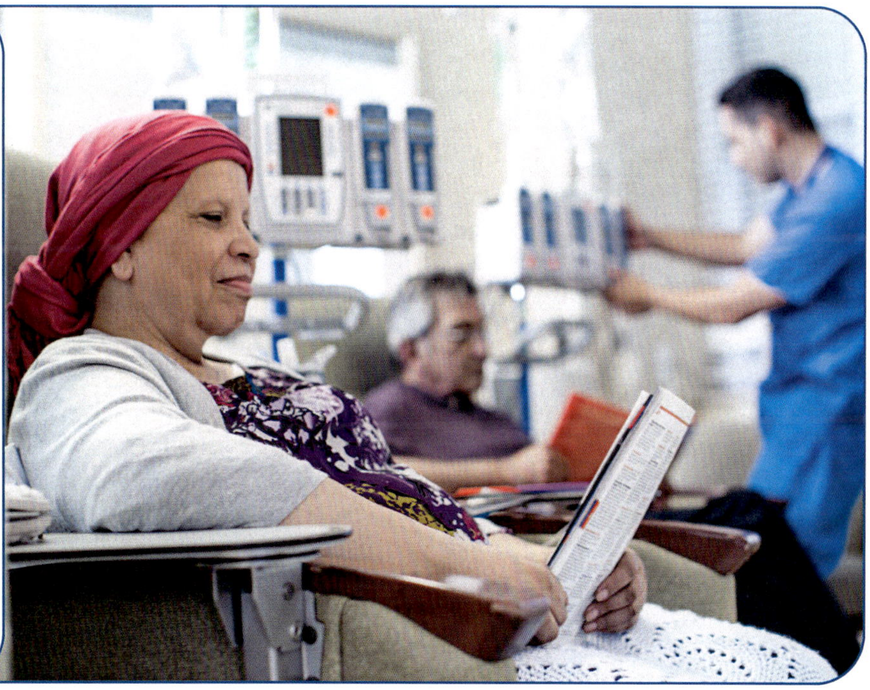

You will not receive chemotherapy every day. Instead, it will be given in cycles of treatment days followed by days of rest. These cycles give your body a chance to recover after receiving chemotherapy.

You will need to go to a treatment center to get chemotherapy. The chemotherapy will be slowly injected into your vein. This is called an infusion. Chemotherapy travels in your bloodstream to treat cancer throughout your body.

Curing lung cancer with chemoradiation

Definitive chemoradiation is a treatment option for some stage 2B and stage 3 cancers.

There are 2 scheduling approaches to deliver chemoradiation:

- **Concurrent chemoradiation** means that chemotherapy and radiation therapy are given at the same time.
- **Sequential chemoradiation** means you will first complete chemotherapy and then receive radiation therapy. This schedule may be followed if concurrent treatment is likely too harmful for you.

Schedule of radiation therapy

Radiation therapy is typically delivered in 30 to 35 small doses, called fractions, over 6 to 7 weeks. For sequential chemoradiation, some people are treated with around 15 higher-dose fractions.

Further details about receiving radiation therapy are described in *Chapter 7: Radiation therapy.*

Chemotherapy options for chemoradiation

Chemotherapy regimens used for chemoradiation are listed in **Guide 12.**

The regimens are grouped by NCCN levels of preference:

- **Preferred therapies** have the most evidence they work better and may be safer than other therapies.
- **Other recommended therapies** may not work quite as well as preferred therapies, but they can still help treat cancer.
- **Therapies used in certain cases** work best for people with specific cancer features or health circumstances.

Consolidation treatment

The goals of consolidation are to bolster the results of treatment and improve the chance of a cure.

There are 2 options for consolidation treatment after definitive concurrent chemoradiation:

- Osimertinib (Tagrisso) for lung cancers **with** an *EGFR* exon 19 deletion or exon 21 L858R mutation
- Durvalumab (Imfinzi) for lung cancers **without** an *EGFR* exon 19 deletion or exon 21 L858R mutation

Osimertinib is a cancer drug called an EGFR kinase inhibitor. EGFR is a cell protein that helps start cell growth. Osimertinib stops the activity of EGFR and, in turn, lowers the number of new cancer cells being made. It is a pill that can be taken at home.

Durvalumab is a cancer drug called an immune checkpoint inhibitor. It works by enabling immune T cells to attack cancer cells. It is given by infusion.

Treatment side effects

Side effects are unwanted health issues caused by treatment. They differ between people based on the type and length of treatment as well as the person.

Side effects from chemotherapy are caused by the death of fast-growing normal cells. Examples include nausea and vomiting, anemia, and hair loss. Side effects are typically worse with concurrent chemoradiation compared with sequential chemoradiation.

Guide 12
Regimens for chemoradiation to treat NSCLC

	Sequential chemoradiation	Concurrent chemoradiation
Adenocarcinoma, large cell carcinoma, and rare cell types	Preferred therapies: • Cisplatin, pemetrexed Other recommended therapies: • Cisplatin, vinorelbine • Cisplatin, etoposide Therapies used in certain cases: • Carboplatin, paclitaxel • Carboplatin, pemetrexed	Preferred therapies: • Carboplatin, pemetrexed • Cisplatin, pemetrexed • Carboplatin, paclitaxel • Cisplatin, etoposide
	Sequential chemoradiation	**Concurrent chemoradiation**
Squamous cell carcinoma	Preferred therapies: • Cisplatin, gemcitabine • Cisplatin, docetaxel Other recommended therapies: • Cisplatin, vinorelbine • Cisplatin, etoposide Therapies used in certain cases: • Carboplatin, paclitaxel • Carboplatin, gemcitabine	Preferred therapies: • Carboplatin, paclitaxel • Cisplatin, etoposide

Immune checkpoint inhibitors can cause your immune cells to attack healthy cells in your body. Side effects include rash, mouth pain, and fatigue.

Management of side effects is discussed in *Chapter 4: Improving life with supportive care.*

What's next?

Once there are no signs of cancer, surveillance is started. Surveillance is ongoing testing for the return of cancer. It is a part of survivorship care. Survivorship care also focuses on the management of long-term and late effects of cancer. To learn more, read *Chapter 9: Survivorship care*.

Key points

- Chemoradiation is a treatment with both chemotherapy and radiation therapy. It may be used to try to cure lung cancer.
- Chemotherapy for lung cancer often consists of a drug made with platinum and one other drug. It is slowly infused into a vein.
- For chemoradiation, chemotherapy and radiation therapy are typically given at the same time, but sometimes chemotherapy is given first.
- More treatment may be received after chemoradiation to improve the chance of a cure. This is called consolidation.

Questions to ask

- How did you decide what type of chemoradiation is best for me?
- What is the schedule, or cycles, of the chemotherapy?
- Do I need consolidation treatment?
- What are the common and serious side effects of my treatments?

9
Survivorship care

64 Monitoring your health

64 Testing for cancer

66 Managing physical and mental effects

66 Addressing social and financial needs

67 Preventing disease

67 What's next

68 Key points

68 Questions to ask

Survivorship care often begins after initial cancer treatment ends. Its focus is on the wide and lasting impact of cancer and its treatment. Survivorship care will help you recover from cancer and prevent disease.

Monitoring your health

When survivorship care starts, it's very important that your health care providers work together to give you ongoing, coordinated care. At this stage, you'll see your primary care provider more often and see non-cancer specialists as well.

NCCN recommends:

- Routine blood pressure, cholesterol, and glucose monitoring
- Routine dental exams
- Bone density testing if needed
- Pulmonary rehabilitation if needed

You will also have follow-up visits with your cancer care team. They will test for cancer and assess for side effects as explained next.

Testing for cancer

While non-small cell lung cancer (NSCLC) can sometimes be cured, it is very important to watch for the return of the cancer. The return of cancer is called a recurrence. It is also important to be checked for other types of cancer.

Pulmonary rehabilitation

As part of survivorship care, you may see more health specialists. People who have chronic obstructive pulmonary disease (COPD) or pulmonary hypertension commonly receive pulmonary rehabilitation. If you had lung surgery, your team may refer to pulmonary rehabilitation.

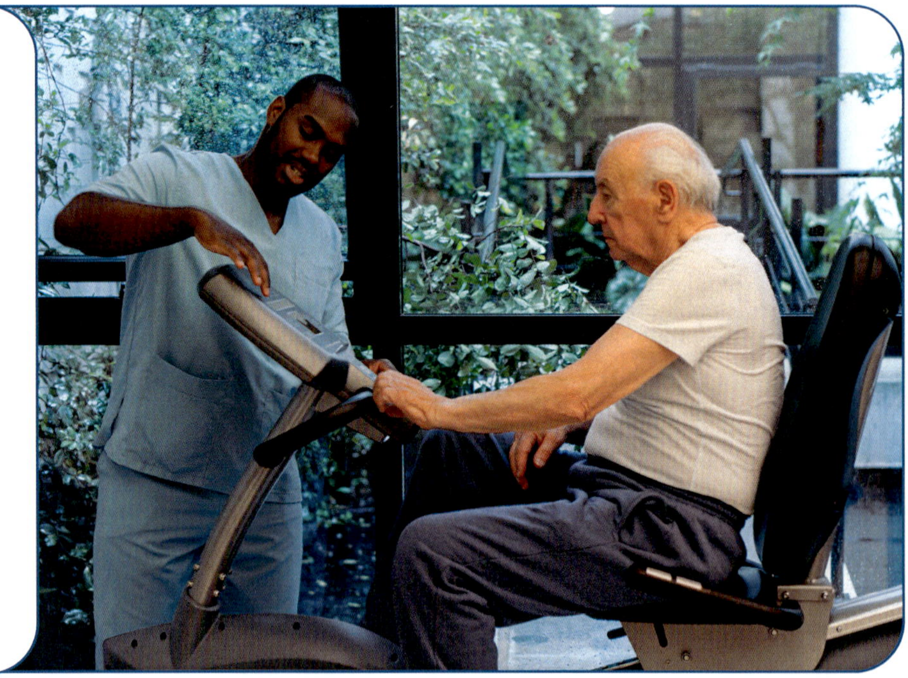

Surveillance for recurrence

Survivorship care includes a schedule of health visits and tests to check for recurrence. These ongoing checkups for recurrence are called surveillance. Surveillance is started when there are no signs of cancer after treatment.

If your care team detects a recurrence early, it will allow for timely treatment. You will need to update your medical history, get physical exams, and undergo computed tomography (CT) scans. Some people may have a magnetic resonance imaging (MRI) scan of their brain. A schedule of surveillance tests is listed in **Guide 13.**

Screening for second cancers

You are at risk for a second cancer. Anyone who has been treated and cured of one lung cancer is at risk for a new lung cancer. Also, a

Guide 13
Surveillance after treatment of non-small cell lung cancer

Stage 1 or stage 2 cancers that were not treated with radiation therapy	Every 6 months for 2 to 3 years, see your care team for a: • Medical history • Physical exam • CT scan of the chest with or without contrast If results are normal, then repeat every year: • Medical history • Physical exam • Low-dose CT scan of the chest
Stage 1 or stage 2 cancers that were treated with radiation therapy **All stage 3 cancers**	Every 3 to 6 months for 3 years, see your care team for a: • Medical history • Physical exam • CT of the chest with or without contrast If results are normal, then repeat every 6 months for 2 years: • Medical history • Physical exam • CT scan of the chest with or without contrast If results remain normal, then repeat every year: • Medical history • Physical exam • Low-dose CT scan of the chest

second cancer is a possible late effect of some cancer treatments.

More information on second cancers is in *NCCN Guidelines for Patients: Survivorship Care for Cancer-Related Late and Long-Term Effects,* available at NCCN.org/patientguidelines and on the NCCN Patient Guides for Cancer app.

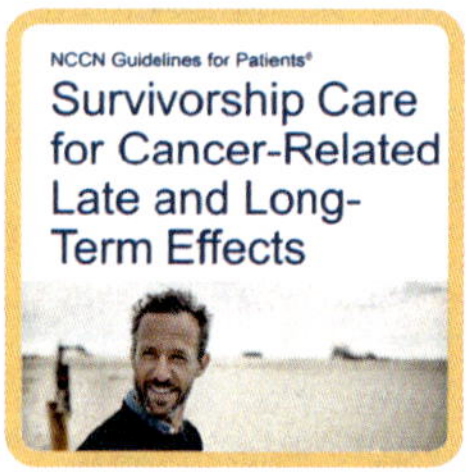

Cancer screening involves routine testing for cancer before its symptoms start. You may enroll in a screening program if you have an average risk for prostate, breast, cervical, colorectal, and skin cancers.

Managing physical and mental effects

As explained in Chapter 4, cancer and its treatment can cause unwanted health issues. These issues are called complications, adverse events, or side effects.

Many side effects of treatment quickly resolve after treatment ends. But during survivorship care, your team will continue to assess for side effects.

Long-term effects start during treatment and persist after treatment is done. Less often, late effects from the cancer or treatment start long after treatment has ended.

NCCN Guidelines for Patients: Survivorship Care for Cancer-Related Late and Long-Term Effects discuss management of many effects, including:

- Heart disease
- Lymphedema
- Chemobrain
- Fatigue and sleep-wake disorders
- Pain
- Distress and mental health

Addressing social and financial needs

You may have social and financial needs during or after lung cancer treatment. As part of survivorship care, your care team will continue to ask you about food, housing, health insurance, and other needs.

A common issue during survivorship is deciding on whether to return to work. Your health care providers can help you. Information on returning to work is in *NCCN Guidelines for Patients: Survivorship Care for Cancer-Related Late and Long-Term Effects.*

Preventing disease

Another part of survivorship care is preventing diseases. This section conveys recommendations from NCCN lung cancer experts.

Immunization shots

Many vaccines safely prevent infections in survivors of lung cancer. You may get the following vaccines as needed:

- Flu shot every year
- COVID-19 vaccine
- Shingles vaccine
- Pneumococcal vaccine with revaccination
- Hepatitis vaccine

Healthy living

It's important for everyone to start or keep a healthy lifestyle —but it's even more important for people who've had cancer. Healthy living may improve your health and well-being. It may also help prevent cancer from returning.

Common goals for healthy living include:

- No smoking
- Being physically active and avoiding inactivity
- Eating healthful foods and drinking little or no alcohol
- Managing body weight to maintain or improve health
- Routine sun protection

More information on preventing poor health can be found in *NCCN Guidelines for Patients: Survivorship Care for Healthy* Living.

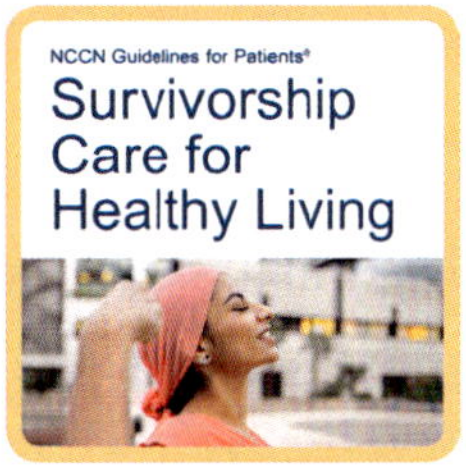

What's next

It's common to have many concerns about cancer. Your care team will support you. More sources of support are listed in *Chapter 10: Other resources.*

I began seeing a therapist during my treatment and I have continued to this day. There are so many thoughts running through your head before, during, and after treatment. It helps to have someone to talk to. A lot of my friends and family don't understand what having cancer is like, so I sought out places where I could talk to survivors. I started going to local support groups and joined several Facebook support groups as well.

Key points

- It's important that your health care providers work together to address all your needs.
- You'll have regular tests to check for a return of lung cancer and for new cancers.
- Your team will assess ongoing side effects as well as new ones at follow-up visits. They will also ask if you have social and financial challenges.
- Healthy living and vaccines may improve your health and prevent disease.

Questions to ask

- How will you coordinate care with my other health care providers?
- How can late side effects be prevented or treated?
- Who can I talk to about help with paying bills, returning to work, and other needs?
- Which vaccines do I need?
- What goals for health living do you recommend for me?

10
Other resources

70 What else to know

70 What else to do

70 Where to get help

71 Questions to ask

Want to learn more? Here's how you can get additional help.

What else to know

This book can help you improve your cancer care. It plainly explains expert recommendations and suggests questions to ask your care team. But it's not the only resource that you have.

You're welcome to receive as much information and help as you need. Many people are interested in learning more about:

- The details of their cancer and treatment
- Finding a care provider who is an expert in lung cancer
- Getting a second opinion
- Being a part of a care team
- Support groups in the community and online

What else to do

Your health care center can help you with next steps. They often have on-site resources to help meet your needs and find answers to your questions. Health care centers can also inform you of resources in your community.

In addition to help from your providers, the resources listed in the next section provide support for many people like yourself. Look through the list and visit the provided websites to learn more about these organizations.

Where to get help

American Lung Association
lung.org/lung-health-diseases/lung-disease-lookup/lung-cancer

Bag It
Bagitcancer.org

Cancer*Care*
Cancercare.org

Cancer Hope Network
cancerhopenetwork.org

Cancer Survivor Care
Cancersurvivorcare.org

Caring Ambassadors Program, Inc.
LungCancerCAP.org

Free Me from Lung Cancer
freemefromlungcancer.org

Go2 Foundation for Lung Cancer
go2foundation.org

Imerman Angels
Imermanangel.org

LiveLung (Dusty Joy Foundation)
dustyjoy.org

LUNGevity
lungevity.org

Lung Cancer Action Network (LungCAN)
lungcan.org

Lung Cancer Research Foundation
lungcancerresearchfoundation.org

National Coalition for Cancer Survivorship
canceradvocacy.org

Triage Cancer
triagecancer.org

Questions to ask

- How do I find a health care provider who's an expert in lung cancer?
- What are the steps to get a second opinion?
- What's my role in making decisions on the best cancer care for me?
- How can I connect with others and build a support system?

Words to know

3D-CRT
Three-dimensional conformal radiation therapy

adenocarcinoma
A cancer of cells that line organs and make fluids or hormones.

biopsy
A procedure that removes fluid or tissue samples to be tested for a disease.

board certified
A status for doctors who finished training and passed exams in a specialized field of medicine.

bronchoscope
A device that is guided down the throat to look inside the airways.

bronchoscopy
A procedure to look inside the airways with a device that is guided down the throat.

cancer screening
Routine testing for cancer in people without symptoms.

cancer stage
A rating of the outlook of a cancer based on its growth and spread.

carcinoma
A cancer of cells that line the inner or outer surfaces of the body.

chemistry profile
A lab test of the amount of 8 chemicals in a sample of blood. Also called metabolic panel.

chemoradiation
A cancer treatment with both cell-killing drugs and high-energy rays.

chemotherapy
Treatment with cancer drugs that kill fast-growing cells.

chest wall
The layer of muscle, bone, and fat that protects the vital organs.

chronic obstructive pulmonary disease (COPD)
Lung damage or too much mucus that makes breathing hard.

clinical stage
The rating of the extent of cancer before treatment is started.

clinical trial
A type of research that assesses how well health tests or treatments work in people.

complete blood count (CBC)
A lab test that measures the parts of the blood.

computed tomography (CT)
A test that uses x-rays from many angles to make a picture of the insides of the body.

contrast
A substance put into your body to make clearer pictures during imaging.

diagnosis
An identification of an illness based on tests.

endobronchial ultrasound (EBUS)
A procedure that takes detailed pictures inside the body with a device guided down the windpipe.

endoscopic ultrasound (EUS)
A procedure that takes detailed pictures inside the body with a device guided down the throat.

esophagus
The tube-shaped organ between the mouth and stomach.

external beam radiation therapy (EBRT)
Radiation therapy received from a machine outside the body.

FDA
Food and Drug Administration

FDG
fluorodeoxyglucose

four-dimensional computed tomography (4D-CT)
A test that makes of video of the inside of your body.

intensity-modulated radiation therapy (IMRT)
Treatment with radiation that uses small beams of different strengths.

invasion
The growth of cancer from where it started into another type of tissue.

large-cell lung carcinoma
A cancer of lung cells that lack features to classify as another type of lung cancer.

lobe
A clearly seen division in an organ.

lobectomy
An operation that removes a whole lobe of an organ.

low-dose computed tomography (LDCT)
A test that uses small amounts of radiation to make pictures of the insides of the body.

lymph node
A small, bean-shaped, disease-fighting structure.

magnetic resonance imaging (MRI)
A test that uses radio waves and powerful magnets to make pictures of the insides of the body.

mediastinoscopy
A procedure in the chest with a device passed through a small cut in the skin.

mediastinum
The area of the chest between the lungs.

medical history
A report of all your health events and medications.

metastasis
The spread of cancer from the first tumor to a new site.

NCCN
National Comprehensive Cancer Network

nodule
A small mass of tissue.

non-small cell lung cancer (NSCLC)
A cancer that starts in lung cells that are not small.

non-solid nodule
A small tissue mass of low density.

part-solid nodule
A small tissue mass with areas of low and high density.

pathologic stage
A rating of the extent of cancer based on tests given after treatment.

pathologist
A doctor who's an expert in testing cells to find disease.

physical exam
A review of the body by a health expert for signs of disease.

pneumonectomy
An operation that removes the entire lung.

positron emission tomography (PET)
A test that uses radioactive material to see the shape and function of body parts.

positron emission tomography/computed tomography (PET/CT)
A test that uses two picture-making methods to show the shape and function of tissue.

postoperative therapy
Treatment that is given after the main treatment to prevent the cancer from returning. also called adjuvant therapy.

preoperative therapy
A cancer treatment that is given before the main treatment. Also called neoadjuvant therapy.

primary tumor
The main mass of a certain type of cancer cell.

prognosis
The likely course and outcome of a disease based on tests.

proton therapy
Radiation therapy that uses protons to treat a disease. Also called hadron therapy.

pulmonary function tests
A set of breathing tests to test the strength of the lungs.

pulmonologist
A doctor who's an expert in lung diseases.

radial endobronchial ultrasound (EBUS) bronchoscopy
A procedure to do work inside the lung with an imaging device guided down the windpipe.

radiation oncologist
A doctor who's an expert in treating cancer with radiation.

radiation therapy
A treatment that uses intense energy to kill cancer cells.

risk factor
Anything that increases the chance of an event.

robot-assisted thoracoscopic surgery (RATS)
A method to perform a surgery called thoracoscopy.

segmentectomy
An operation that removes a large part of a lobe.

side effect
An unhealthy or unpleasant physical or emotional response to treatment.

sleeve lobectomy
An operation to remove an entire lobe and part of the bronchus.

solid nodule
A small mass of tissue of high density.

squamous cell carcinoma
A type of cancer of thin and flat cells that line the surface of organs.

stereotactic ablative radiotherapy (SABR)
Treatment with high-dose radiation within one or a few sessions. Also called stereotactic body radiation therapy.

superior sulcus tumor
A mass of cancer cells that starts at the top of the lung and easily grows into the chest wall.

supportive care
Cancer care that includes symptom relief but not cancer treatment. Also sometimes called palliative care.

surgery
An operation to remove or repair a part of the body.

surgical margin
The normal-looking tissue around a tumor that was removed during an operation.

survivorship care
Interventions to improve the health and well-being of people who have or had cancer.

targeted therapy
A drug treatment that impedes the growth process specific to cancer cells.

thoracic radiologist
A doctor who's an expert in reading imaging tests of the chest.

thoracic surgeon
A doctor who's an expert in operating on organs inside the chest.

thoracoscopy
A procedure to do work in the chest with a device passed through a small cut in the skin.

three-dimensional conformal radiation therapy (3D-CRT)
A treatment with radiation that uses beams matched to the shape of the tumor.

transthoracic needle aspiration (TTNA)
A procedure that removes tissue samples with a thin needle guided through the ribs.

ultrasound
A test that uses sound waves to take pictures of the inside of the body.

video-assisted thoracoscopic surgery (VATS)
A method to perform a surgery called thoracoscopy.

wedge resection
An operation that removes a small part of a lobe.

NCCN Contributors

This patient guide is based on the NCCN Clinical Practice Guidelines in Oncology (NCCN Guidelines®) for Non-Small Cell Lung Cancer, Version 3.2025. It was adapted, reviewed, and published with help from the following people:

Dorothy A. Shead, MS
Senior Director
Patient Information Operations

Laura J. Hanisch, PsyD
Patient Information Program Manager

Susan Kidney
Senior Graphic Design Specialist

The NCCN Clinical Practice Guidelines in Oncology (NCCN Guidelines®) for Non-Small Cell Lung Cancer, Version 3.2025 were developed by the following NCCN Panel Members:

Gregory J. Riely, MD, PhD/Chair
Memorial Sloan Kettering Cancer Center

Douglas E. Wood, MD/Vice Chair
Fred Hutchinson Cancer Center

Dara L. Aisner, MD, PhD
University of Colorado Cancer Center

Wallace Akerley, MD
Huntsman Cancer Institute at the University of Utah

Jessica R. Bauman, MD
Fox Chase Cancer Center

Ankit Bharat, MD
Robert H. Lurie Comprehensive Cancer Center of Northwestern University

Joe Y. Chang, MD, PhD
The University of Texas MD Anderson Cancer Center

Lucian R. Chirieac, MD
Dana-Farber/Brigham and Women's Cancer Center

Malcolm DeCamp, MD
University of Wisconsin Carbone Cancer Center

Aakash Desai, MD, MPH
O'Neal Comprehensive Cancer Center at UAB

Thomas J. Dilling, MD, MS
Moffitt Cancer Center

Jonathan Dowell, MD
UT Southwestern Simmons Comprehensive Cancer Center

Gregory A. Durm, MD, MS
Indiana University Melvin and Bren Simon Comprehensive Cancer Center

Scott Gettinger, MD
Yale Cancer Center/Smilow Cancer Hospital

Travis E. Grotz, MD
Mayo Clinic Comprehensive Cancer Center

Matthew A. Gubens, MD, MS
UCSF Helen Diller Family Comprehensive Cancer Center

Aditya Juloori, MD
The UChicago Medicine Comprehensive Cancer Center

Rudy P. Lackner, MD
Fred & Pamela Buffett Cancer Center

Michael Lanuti, MD
Mass General Cancer Center

Jules Lin, MD
University of Michigan Rogel Cancer Center

Billy W. Loo, Jr, MD, PhD
Stanford Cancer Institute

Christine M. Lovly, MD, PhD
Vanderbilt-Ingram Cancer Center

Fabien Maldonado, MD
Vanderbilt-Ingram Cancer Center

Daniel Morgensztern, MD
Siteman Cancer Center at Barnes-Jewish Hospital and Washington University School of Medicine

Trey C. Mullikin, MD
Duke Cancer Institute

Thomas Ng, MD
The University of Tennessee Health Science Center

*Dawn Owen, MD, PhD
Mayo Clinic Comprehensive Cancer Center

Dwight H. Owen, MD, MSc
The Ohio State University Comprehensive Cancer Center - James Cancer Hospital and Solove Research Institute

Sandip P. Patel, MD
UC San Diego Moores Cancer Center

Tejas Patil, MD
University of Colorado Cancer Center

Patricio M. Polanco, MD
UT Southwestern Simmons Comprehensive Cancer Center

Jonathan Riess, MD
UC Davis Comprehensive Cancer Center

*Theresa A. Shapiro, MD, PhD
Johns Hopkins Kimmel Cancer Center

Aditi P. Singh, MD
Abramson Cancer Center at the University of Pennsylvania

James Stevenson, MD/Lead
Case Comprehensive Cancer Center/ University Hospitals Seidman Cancer Center and Cleveland Clinic Taussig Cancer Institute

Alda Tam, MD
The University of Texas MD Anderson Cancer Center

*Tawee Tanvetyanon, MD, MPH
Moffitt Cancer Center

Jane Yanagawa, MD
UCLA Jonsson Comprehensive Cancer Center

Stephen C. Yang, MD
Johns Hopkins Kimmel Cancer Center

Edwin Yau, MD, PhD
Roswell Park Comprehensive Cancer Center

NCCN

Kristina Gregory, RN, MSN
Senior Vice President, Clinical Information Programs

Lisa Hang, PhD
Oncology Scientist/Senior Medical Writer

* Reviewed this patient guide. For disclosures, visit NCCN.org/disclosures.

NCCN Cancer Centers

Abramson Cancer Center
at the University of Pennsylvania
Philadelphia, Pennsylvania
800.789.7366 • pennmedicine.org/cancer

Case Comprehensive Cancer Center/
University Hospitals Seidman Cancer Center and
Cleveland Clinic Taussig Cancer Institute
Cleveland, Ohio
UH Seidman Cancer Center
800.641.2422 • uhhospitals.org/services/cancer-services
CC Taussig Cancer Institute
866.223.8100 • my.clevelandclinic.org/departments/cancer
Case CCC
216.844.8797 • case.edu/cancer

City of Hope National Medical Center
Duarte, California
800.826.4673 • cityofhope.org

Dana-Farber/Brigham and Women's Cancer Center |
Mass General Cancer Center
Boston, Massachusetts
877.442.3324 • youhaveus.org
617.726.5130 • massgeneral.org/cancer-center

Duke Cancer Institute
Durham, North Carolina
888.275.3853 • dukecancerinstitute.org

Fox Chase Cancer Center
Philadelphia, Pennsylvania
888.369.2427 • foxchase.org

Fred & Pamela Buffett Cancer Center
Omaha, Nebraska
402.559.5600 • unmc.edu/cancercenter

Fred Hutchinson Cancer Center
Seattle, Washington
206.667.5000 • fredhutch.org

Huntsman Cancer Institute at the University of Utah
Salt Lake City, Utah
800.824.2073 • healthcare.utah.edu/huntsmancancerinstitute

Indiana University Melvin and Bren Simon
Comprehensive Cancer Center
Indianapolis, Indiana
888.600.4822 • www.cancer.iu.edu

Johns Hopkins Kimmel Cancer Center
Baltimore, Maryland
410.955.8964
www.hopkinskimmelcancercenter.org

Mayo Clinic Comprehensive Cancer Center
Phoenix/Scottsdale, Arizona
Jacksonville, Florida
Rochester, Minnesota
480.301.8000 • Arizona
904.953.0853 • Florida
507.538.3270 • Minnesota
mayoclinic.org/cancercenter

Memorial Sloan Kettering Cancer Center
New York, New York
800.525.2225 • mskcc.org

Moffitt Cancer Center
Tampa, Florida
888.663.3488 • moffitt.org

O'Neal Comprehensive Cancer Center at UAB
Birmingham, Alabama
800.822.0933 • uab.edu/onealcancercenter

Robert H. Lurie Comprehensive Cancer Center
of Northwestern University
Chicago, Illinois
866.587.4322 • cancer.northwestern.edu

Roswell Park Comprehensive Cancer Center
Buffalo, New York
877.275.7724 • roswellpark.org

Siteman Cancer Center at Barnes-Jewish Hospital
and Washington University School of Medicine
St. Louis, Missouri
800.600.3606 • siteman.wustl.edu

St. Jude Children's Research Hospital/
The University of Tennessee Health Science Center
Memphis, Tennessee
866.278.5833 • stjude.org
901.448.5500 • uthsc.edu

Stanford Cancer Institute
Stanford, California
877.668.7535 • cancer.stanford.edu

The Ohio State University Comprehensive Cancer Center -
James Cancer Hospital and Solove Research Institute
Columbus, Ohio
800.293.5066 • cancer.osu.edu

The UChicago Medicine Comprehensive Cancer Center
Chicago, Illinois
773.702.1000 • uchicagomedicine.org/cancer

The University of Texas MD Anderson Cancer Center
Houston, Texas
844.269.5922 • mdanderson.org

UC Davis Comprehensive Cancer Center
Sacramento, California
916.734.5959 • 800.770.9261
health.ucdavis.edu/cancer

UC San Diego Moores Cancer Center
La Jolla, California
858.822.6100 • cancer.ucsd.edu

UCLA Jonsson Comprehensive Cancer Center
Los Angeles, California
310.825.5268 • uclahealth.org/cancer

UCSF Helen Diller Family
Comprehensive Cancer Center
San Francisco, California
800.689.8273 • cancer.ucsf.edu

University of Colorado Cancer Center
Aurora, Colorado
720.848.0300 • coloradocancercenter.org

University of Michigan Rogel Cancer Center
Ann Arbor, Michigan
800.865.1125 • rogelcancercenter.org

University of Wisconsin Carbone Cancer Center
Madison, Wisconsin
608.265.1700 • uwhealth.org/cancer

UT Southwestern Simmons
Comprehensive Cancer Center
Dallas, Texas
214.648.3111 • utsouthwestern.edu/simmons

Vanderbilt-Ingram Cancer Center
Nashville, Tennessee
877.936.8422 • vicc.org

Yale Cancer Center/Smilow Cancer Hospital
New Haven, Connecticut
855.4.SMILOW • yalecancercenter.org

share with us.

Take our survey and help make the NCCN Guidelines for Patients better for everyone!

NCCN.org/patients/comments

Index

biopsy 9, 12–16, 23–24

bronchoscopy 16, 23–24

cancer stage 7, 21, 33, 36,

chemoradiation 33, 43, 49, 59–61

chemotherapy 30, 43–45, 49–50, 55–56, 59–61

clinical trial 38–39

imaging 9, 11–12, 22–23

immune checkpoint inhibitors 30, 43–44

low-dose computed tomography 12, 65

medical history 20–21, 65

NCCN Cancer Centers 78

NCCN Contributors 77

pathology report 16

physical exam 21, 65

postoperative therapy 44, 49–50, 55–56

preoperative therapy 44–46

radiation therapy 11, 30, 33, 42–43, 49, 54–56, 59–60

risk factor 10–11

second opinion 70

side effect 28–30, 43, 48, 56, 61–62

superior sulcus tumor 22, 45

supportive care 6, 28–30

surgery 16, 23–25, 33, 36–37, 42–48, 54, 59, 64

survivorship care 64–67

targeted therapy 43, 49–50

Made in United States
North Haven, CT
24 January 2026

87101522R00046